Patients Beyond Borders™
Thailand Edition

Everybody's Guide to Affordable,
World-Class Medical Tourism

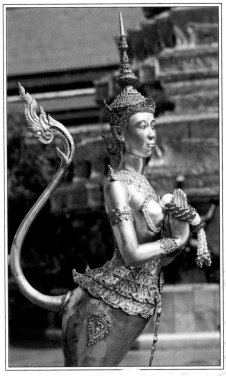

Josef Woodman

MEDIA

...eyondborders.com

N Thailand

The Kingdom of Thailand is an independent country nestled in the heart of Southeast Asia, bordered to the north by Lao PDR (Laos) and Myanmar (Burma), east by Lao PDR and Cambodia, south by the Gulf of Thailand and Malaysia, and west by the Andaman Sea and Myanmar. Bangkok is Thailand's capital and biggest city, and also its political, commercial, industrial, and cultural center. Bangkok and its environs have a population of more than 10.1 million.

Thailand is the world's fiftieth largest country, with a land mass of around 200,000 square miles (nearly 518,000 square kilometers), and is the world's twentieth largest country in terms of population. The local climate is tropical, with predictable monsoon seasons: a warm southwest monsoon from mid-May to September, and a cooler northeast monsoon from November to February. Thailand's southern isthmus is nearly always hot and humid.

Tourism is one of Thailand's largest industries; nearly 15 million visited the kingdom in 2008. Thailand offers a great variety of attractions, including temples, World Heritage sites, archaeological sites, cultural museums, exceptional flora and bird life, hill tribes, marine parks and diving destinations, sandy beaches, hundreds of tropical islands, and varied nightlife.

The Andaman Sea is considered one of Thailand's most precious natural resources, as it is Asia's most popular and luxurious resort area. Phuket, Krabi, Ranong, Phang Nga, Trang, and other lush islands all lie along the coast of the Andaman Sea. Despite the 2004 tsunami, these destinations continue to welcome tourists from all over Asia and the world.

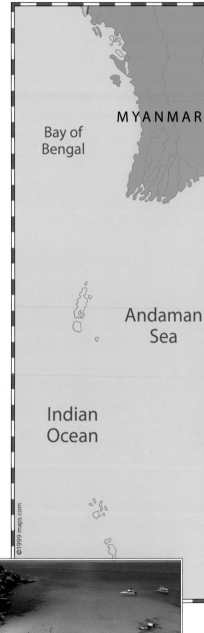

Bay of Bengal

MYANMAR

Andaman Sea

Indian Ocean

©1999 maps.com

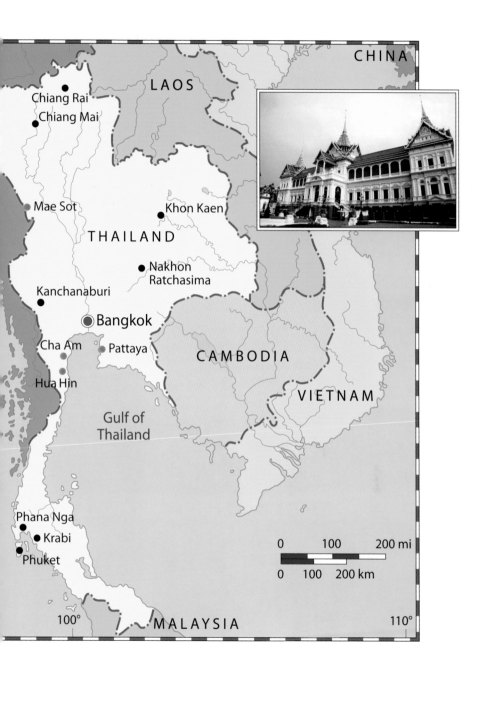

CHINA

LAOS

● Chiang Rai
● Chiang Mai

● Mae Sot

THAILAND

● Khon Kaen

● Nakhon
Ratchasima

Kanchanaburi
●

⦿ Bangkok

Cha Am ●
● Pattaya

CAMBODIA

Hua Hin ●

Gulf of
Thailand

VIETNAM

● Phana Nga
● Krabi
● Phuket

0   100   200 mi

0   100   200 km

100°   110°

MALAYSIA

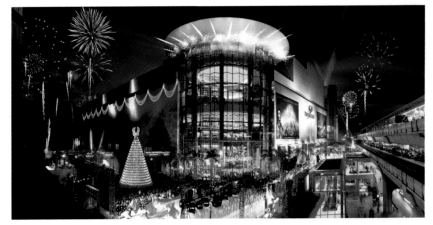

Siam Paragon

Bangkok
is the
cosmopolitan
heart of
Thailand.

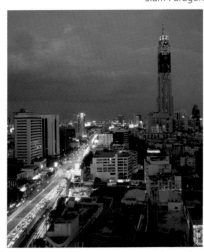

Bangkok at night

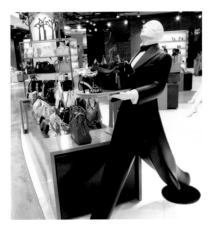

Upscale shops and boutiques await

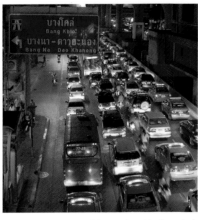

A busy street in Bangkok

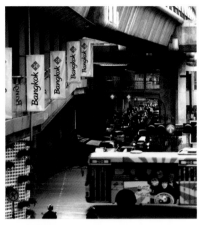

Bangkok street scene

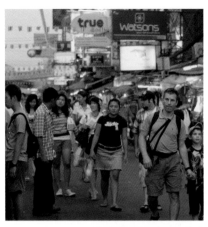

Khao San Road, Bangkok

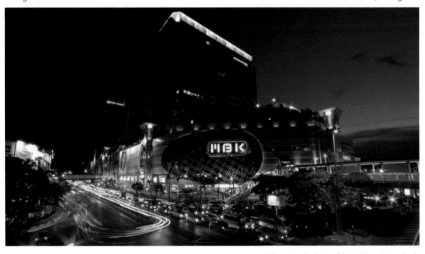

The city lights of bustling Bangkok

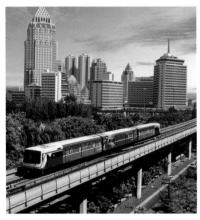

Bangkok Sky Train

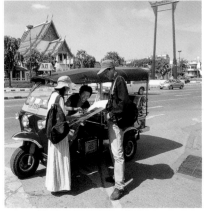

Tuk-tuks are popular in the city

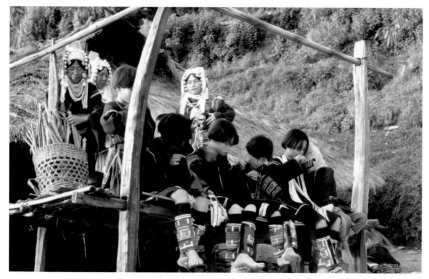

Hilltribe People

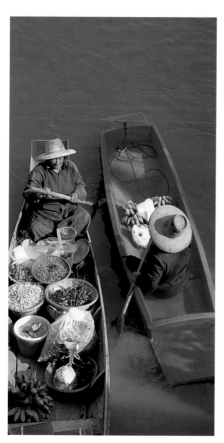

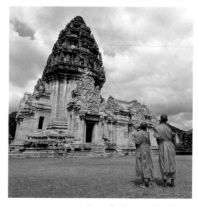

Temple in rural Thailand

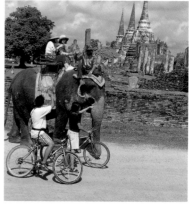

Khlong tour, Bangkok

Popular elephant rides

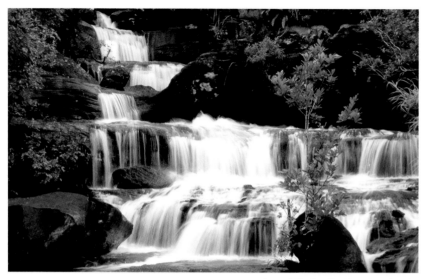
One of Thailand's 48 national parks

Enjoy the
flora and
fauna of
Thailand's
national parks.

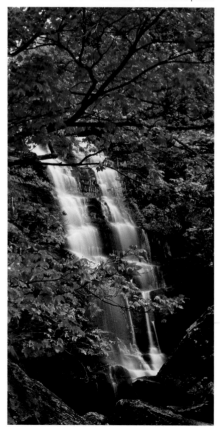

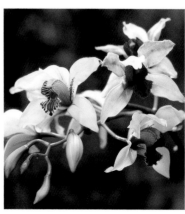
Orchids abound in rural Thailand

Khun Phong Waterfall

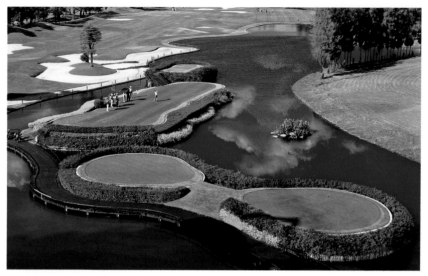
Summit Windmill Golf Club

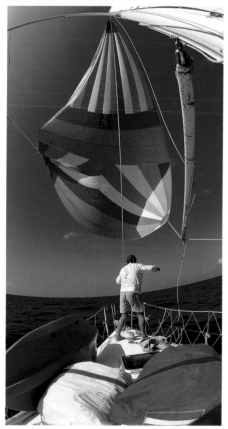

From golfing
to sailing,
Thailand
offers
something for
everybody.

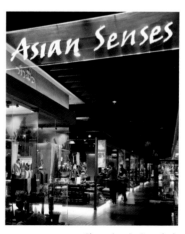

Sailing the Gulf

Shopping in Bangkok

"A useful new book on this topic . . ."

—*Savvy Senior*

"I am considering elective surgery and this was a great compendium of information scattered all over the Internet."

—Amy Tupper (Sanford, NC)

"I spent a lot of time on the Internet trying to research this topic on my own and looking for certain procedures (mainly dental and cosmetic surgery). I wound up getting dental work done in Mexico at a facility reviewed in [*Patients Beyond Borders*] and am happy with my experience. I recommend this book to anyone even remotely considering foreign medical travel."

— K. Williamson (Los Lunas, NM)

"If the American healthcare system is not completely broken, it is certainly dysfunctional: 47 million people have no health coverage, and 130 million have no dental insurance. As baby boomers age into more medical problems with spotty coverage and would prefer not to deplete their retirement savings, they are looking at all available options."

—*Financial Times*

"A must-read for those considering medical tourism . . ."

—*ABC News*

"A practical guide to planning a medical trip . . ."

—*Washington Post*

Patients Beyond Borders Series™

Patients Beyond Borders™
Thailand Edition

Everybody's Guide to Affordable,
World-Class Medical Tourism

Josef Woodman

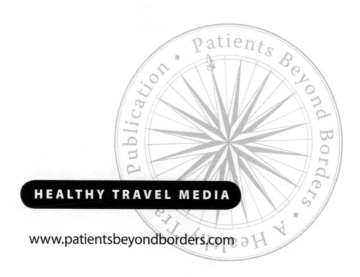

HEALTHY TRAVEL MEDIA

www.patientsbeyondborders.com

PATIENTS BEYOND BORDERS: THAILAND EDITION
Everybody's Guide to Affordable, World-Class Medical Tourism

Copyright © 2009 by Josef Woodman

ISBN 13: 978-0-9823361-2-0

Cover Art and Page Design: Anne Winslow
Developmental Editing: Faith Brynie
Production Coordination: Budget-Smart Company, Ltd.
Copyediting: Kate Johnson
Proofreading: Barbara Resch
Indexing: Madge Walls
Color Layout: Judy Orchard
Typesetting and Production: Copperline Book Services
POD Printing: United Book Press
Offset Printing: C & C Offset Printers

Printed in the USA and the People's Republic of China

Healthy Travel Media
P.O. Box 17057
Chapel Hill, NC 27516
919 370.7380
info@patientsbeyondborders.com
www.patientsbeyondborders.com

To All the Dedicated Healthcare Workers of Thailand

ACKNOWLEDGMENTS

BY THE TIME this book is published, *Patients Beyond Borders: Thailand Edition* will have been nearly three years in the making. In pondering the many individuals and organizations that figured in this long and rewarding journey, I'm glad I had the opportunity to read John Burdett's brilliant "Bangkok" series, which confronts the reader with the challenges of initiating, negotiating, and completing an undertaking as complex as a book in a town so elaborately intricate as Bangkok. I learned the American way isn't always the shortest distance between two timelines, that even concrete, linear projects can be driven by spirits and a certain magic that often escapes our understanding.

A heartfelt thanks goes out to the many institutions that enthusiastically supported and sponsored this project from the beginning. The Tourism Authority of Thailand (TAT) played a major role, and I greatly appreciate the early support of Khun Srisuda Wanapinyosak and Khun Juthaporn Rerngronasa, without whose sustained efforts this effort would not have come to fruition. Thanks also to Khun Phornsiri Manoharn, formerly the governor of TAT and now the chairperson of the Pacific Asia Travel Association, who early in the project's development saw the importance of inbound medical travel to Thailand's tourism industry.

A number of early boosters on the provider side played key roles as well: thanks to Curt Schroeder, Mack Banner, and Ken Mays for their early vision and input; to Peter Morely for his tireless dedication to the international patient; and many thanks to Dr. Somkiet Chuapetcharasopon for his role as unofficial project emissary in the early days. Beatrice Venturi: you are a gem—how you juggle it all never ceases to amaze me!

Special thanks to Dr. Chatree Duangnet and Dr. Veerachat Petpisit for their last-minute heroics, and to the many individuals at Samitivej who also contributed their resources to the project.

A huge note of gratitude is in order to Wendy Sirisampanth and his team at Budget-Smart. Wendy successfully negotiated the occasionally choppy waters across geographical—and sometimes cultural—distance, to bring this worthy project to completion. Many thanks, Wendy, for helping me understand "the Thai way."

Finally, my appreciation to the editors, proofreaders, and indexer who made the Thailand Edition possible. Special thanks to our editorial director and developmental editor, Faith Brynie, who crafted the manuscript; copyeditor Kate Johnson, who polished the pages and did them proud; and typesetter Nicki Florence, who put in the extra time and effort to get the color pages just right.

Josef Woodman
Chapel Hill, NC
2009

Contents

PART TWO: THAILAND'S MOST POPULAR MEDICAL DESTINATIONS

PART THREE: SPA DESTINATIONS IN THE LAND OF SMILES

PART FOUR: TRAVELING IN THAILAND

PART FIVE: RESOURCES AND REFERENCES

SOME YEARS BACK, shortly after the first edition of *Patients Beyond Borders* was published, I departed from the beautiful island of Phuket on a sorely needed ten-day overland trip to Bangkok. The ride took me along Thailand's breathtaking mountains and coastlines; I eventually hopped the famed Eastern & Oriental Express, which took me a hundred years back, through the peaceful heart of Thailand's rice country and along the lovely hills of Myanmar to the west. I stopped for the weekend in the old diving town of Chumphon and spent two days in the unforgettable temple town of Phetchaburi before turning eastward into bustling Bangkok.

Thailand is truly "the Land of Smiles." Whether in a five-star Hilton or a funky hill-town stopover, I was always greeted with unending, impeccable hospitality—the type of service that can only come from the heart.

Thailand's reputation for incomparable hospitality extends to its medical services as well. Not only is the country's healthcare system one of the best in Asia, but a patient in one of Thailand's many international hospitals can count on the quality of personal service one would expect in a fine hotel.

As the US healthcare system continues to deteriorate, I have become acutely aware of the important relationship between quality of care and customer service. Good food makes for faster recovery. Pleasant, quiet surroundings make for lower stress levels. Lower patient-practitioner ratios help reduce post-op complications and enforce patient compliance. The list goes on, and Thailand's top hospitals have as much as written the operating manual for excellence in medical care and patient services.

Thailand is known as the birthplace of contemporary medical tourism. More than a million foreign patients visit its public and private hospitals every year, and Thailand is home to the world's largest international hospital in terms of patient visits. Complementing the country's excellent internal quality-assurance and accreditation infrastructure are seven Joint Commission International (JCI)–accredited hospitals, along with one of Asia's largest populations of Western-trained physicians, surgeons, and administrators. One Thai hospital boasts more than 200 American board–certified physicians, and at one time Thailand had more computerized tomography scanning equipment per capita than the UK! Surgical success rates among its JCI-accredited facilities compare favorably with those in the US, and each year new procedures and technologies arrive as part of the international patient's menu of healthcare choices. I hope you'll take the time to read our thumbnail history of Thailand's healthcare system, beginning on page 65, then thumb through the profiles of its many leading facilities.

As wellness and preventive care finally become a part of the Western medical vernacular, informed healthcare consumers will quickly discover the benefits of Thailand's rich history as a spa and traditional medicine destination. Nearly 600 spas and wellness resorts—many of them medically supervised—welcome more than 2 million foreign visitors every year. And

Thailand's renowned traditional medicine is fast becoming more accessible to the consumer, with 28 approved herbal remedies now on the market.

As you read through these pages, I hope you'll gain a new appreciation of the important relationship between the clinical medical procedure and the total healing experience. At the forefront of new approaches to medical care, preventive care, recuperation, and recovery—Thailand is light-years ahead of its Western counterparts. As new chapters are written into the global healthcare operating manual, I am quite sure Thailand will figure prominently as a leader and catalyst for change.

Josef Woodman
October 2009

Introduction

If you're holding this copy of *Patients Beyond Borders: Thailand
Edition* in your hands, you probably already know that you need a
medical procedure, and perhaps you are considering an affordable,
trustworthy alternative to care in your own country. As you can
see, this is a specialty volume in the *Patients Beyond Borders* series,
profiling the Kingdom of Thailand as a healthcare destination. It is
intended for those who already have (more or less) a diagnosis and
already know (more or less) what treatment they need.

This edition doesn't provide the breadth of general information
about medical travel that you'll find in our larger book, *Patients
Beyond Borders: Everybody's Guide to Affordable, World-Class
Medical Travel*, now in its Second Edition. Instead, this volume
first offers an overview of the questions you need to answer before you commit to medical travel; then, most of its pages are de-
voted to describing the best places in Thailand to find excellent
treatment and care. It also contains information on health travel

agents who can help you make the necessary arrangements in Thailand at a reasonable price.

The Phenomenon of Medical Travel

In the last three years, I have traveled to 22 countries and visited more than 140 hospitals, talking to surgeons, healthcare administrators, and their patients. Health travelers are often pleasantly surprised at the quality of care, the prices, and the all-around good experience of their medical travel abroad. As we contemplate our options in an overburdened healthcare environment, many of us will eventually find ourselves seeking alternatives to costly treatments—either for ourselves or for our loved ones. Healthcare consumers everywhere are in the midst of a global shift in medical services. In a few short years, big government investment, corporate partnerships, and increased media attention have spawned a new industry, medical tourism, bringing with it a host of encouraging new choices.

This new phenomenon of medical tourism—or international health travel—has recently received a good deal of wide-eyed attention. While one newspaper or blog giddily touts the fun 'n sun side of treatment abroad, another issues dire warnings about filthy hospitals, shady treatment practices, and procedures gone bad. As with most things in life, the truth lies somewhere in between. When I speak to interviewers and reporters, I try to emphasize that "medical tourism" is a misnomer. Medical travel is not a vacation. Unlike some other books on medical travel, this one focuses more on your health than on your recreational preferences. Business travelers don't consider themselves tourists; neither should you. This book will help you think about the "business" of health travel.

Patients Beyond Borders: Thailand Edition isn't a guide to medical diagnosis and treatment, nor does it provide medical advice on specific treatments or caregiver referrals. Your condition, diagnosis, treatment options, and travel preferences are unique, and only you—in consultation with your physician and loved ones—can determine the best course of action. Should you decide to go abroad for treatment, we provide a wealth of resources and tools to help you become an informed medical traveler, so you can have the best possible travel experience and treatment your money can buy.

My research, including countless interviews, has convinced me that with diligence, perseverance, and good information, patients considering traveling to Thailand or any other country for treatment indeed have legitimate, safe choices, not to mention an opportunity to save thousands of dollars over the same treatment in their home country. Hundreds of patients who have returned from successful treatment overseas provide overwhelmingly positive feedback. They have persuaded me to write this series of impartial, scrutinizing guides to treatment options abroad.

Why Cross Borders for Medical Care?

Cost savings. Depending upon the country and type of treatment, uninsured and underinsured patients as well as those seeking elective care can save 15–85 percent of the cost of treatment in their home country. For example, a knee surgery that costs $43,000 in the US may cost (depending on the doctors and facilities) US$10,000 in Thailand, including your hospital stay.

Better quality care. Veteran health travelers know that facilities, instrumentation, and customer service in treatment centers abroad often equal or exceed those found in their own country.

Excluded treatments. Many people don't have health insurance. Even if you do, your policy may exclude a variety of conditions and treatments. You, the policyholder, must pay these expenses out of pocket, so having the procedure in another country where it's more affordable makes economic sense.

Specialty treatments. Some procedures not available in your home country are available abroad. Some procedures that are widely practiced in certain parts of the world have not yet been approved in others, or they have been approved so recently that their availability remains spotty.

Shorter waiting periods. For decades, thousands of Canadian and British subscribers to universal, "free" healthcare plans have endured waits as long as two years for established procedures. Patients living in other countries with socialized medicine are beginning to experience longer waits as well. Some patients figure it's better to pay out of pocket to get out of pain or halt a deteriorating condition than to suffer the anxiety and frustration of waiting for a far-future appointment and other medical uncertainties.

More "inpatient-friendly." Health insurance companies apply significant pressure on hospitals to move patients out of those costly beds as quickly as possible, sometimes before they are ready. In Thailand and many other medical travel destinations, care is taken to ensure that patients are discharged only at the appropriate time and no sooner. Furthermore, staff-to-patient ratios are usually higher abroad, while hospital-borne infection rates are often lower.

The lure of the new and different. Although traveling abroad for medical care can often be challenging, many patients welcome the chance to blaze a trail, and they find the hospitality and creature comforts often offered abroad to be a welcome relief from the sterile, impersonal hospital environments so frequently encountered at home.

Safety and Security

The overriding concern of many patients new to global health travel is safety. That's understandable. Stories of wars, terrorist plots, roadside bombings, subway gassings, mad snipers, and military coups dominate the news. Obviously, we live in a troubled world. Yet, this fact remains: of the more than 3 million patients who traveled overseas for medical treatment in the last five years, we know of no individual who has died as a result of violence or hostility.

In truth, most health travelers are usually quite sheltered. They're chauffeured from the airport to the hospital or hotel, personally driven to consultations, given their meals in their rooms, and chauffeured back to the airport when it's time to go home. US citizens who are concerned about traveling abroad can check the US Department of State's travel advisories at http://travel.state.gov/travel/cis_pa_tw/tw/tw_1764.html. Similar information services are available in other countries.

How to Use This Book

Before you dive into Part Two, please review the checklists and sidebars in **Part One, "Reminders for the Savvy, Informed Medical Traveler."** A shortened version of the more complete information in *Patients Beyond Borders: Second Edition*, it gives you some of the tools you'll need to do your research and make an informed decision. You'll find the following in Part One:

Chapter One: Dos and Don'ts for the Smart Health Traveler

Chapter Two: *Patients Beyond Borders* Budget Planner

Chapter Three: Checklists for Health Travel

> **Checklist 1: Should I Consult a Health Travel Planner?**
>
> **Checklist 2: How Can a Health Travel Planner Help Me?**
>
> **Checklist 3: What Do I Need to Do Ahead of Time?**
>
> **Checklist 4: What Should I Pack?**
>
> **Checklist 5: What Should I Do Just Before and During My Trip?**
>
> **Checklist 6: What Do I Do After My Procedure?**
>
> **Checklist 7: What Does My Travel Companion Need to Do?**

Part Two, "Thailand's Most Popular Medical Destinations," provides a brief overview of healthcare in Thailand today, and profiles 18 prominent healthcare facilities as well as several health travel agencies that serve medical travelers to Thailand. Each entry provides contact information along with a rundown on available services and history of care.

Part Three, "Spa Destinations in the Land of Smiles," describes 21 spas in Thailand that are popular with medical travelers. You may want to book some time in one of them before your medical procedure or afterward, during your recovery. Spas can promote healing—both mental and physical—so they are worth considering if you have the time and the budget.

Part Four, "Traveling in Thailand," provides details on everything from time zones to visas—basic, practical information you'll need to plan your trip. It also describes a number of the sights and experiences to be enjoyed in Thailand.

Part Five, "Resources and References," offers additional sources of travel information and helpful links, plus a glossary of commonly used medical terms.

As you work your way through decision-making and subsequent planning, remember that you're following in the footsteps of hundreds of thousands of health travelers who have made the journey before you. The vast majority have returned home successfully treated, with money to spare in their savings accounts. Still, the process—particularly in the early planning—can be daunting, frustrating, and even a little scary. Every health traveler I've interviewed experienced "the Big Fear" at one time or another. Healthcare abroad is not for everyone, and part of being a smart consumer is evaluating all the impartial data available before making an informed decision. If you accomplish that in reading *Patients Beyond Borders: Thailand Edition*, I've achieved my goal. Let's get started.

PART ONE

Reminders for the Savvy, Informed Medical Traveler

Much of the advice here in Part One is covered in greater detail in *Patients Beyond Borders: Second Edition*. Consider the following three chapters a capsule summary of essential information, sprinkled with practical advice that will help reduce the number of inevitable "gotchas" that health travelers encounter. You may want your travel companion or family members to read this section, along with the book's Introduction, so they can gain a better understanding of medical travel.

Dos and Don'ts
for the Smart Health Traveler

BEFORE YOUR TRIP

✔ *Do* plan ahead.

The farther in advance you plan, the more likely you are to get the best doctors, the lowest airfares, and the best availability and rates on hotels, particularly if you'll be traveling at peak tourist season for your destination country—in Thailand, that's November through March. If possible, begin planning at least three months prior to your expected departure date. If you're concerned about having to change plans, *do* be sure to confirm cancellation policies with airlines, hotels, and travel agents.

✔ *Do* be sure about your diagnosis and treatment needs.

The more you know about the treatment you're seeking, the easier your search for a physician will be. *Do* work closely with your local doctor or medical specialist, and make sure you obtain exact recommendations—in writing, if possible. If you lack confidence in your doctor's diagnosis, seek a second opinion.

✔ *Do* research your in-country doctor thoroughly.

This is the most important step of all. When you've narrowed your search to two or three physicians, invest some time and money in personal telephone interviews, either directly with your candidate doctors or through your health travel planning agency. *Don't* be afraid to ask questions, lots of them, until you feel comfortable that you have chosen a competent physician.

✘ *Don't* rely completely on the Internet for your research.

While it's okay to use the Web for your initial research, *don't* assume that sponsored Web sites offer complete and accurate information. Cross-check your online findings against referrals, articles in leading newspapers and magazines, word of mouth, and your health travel agent.

✔ *Do* consider traveling with a companion.

Many health travelers say they wouldn't go without a close friend or family member by their side. Your travel companion can help you every step of the way. With luck, your companion may even enjoy the trip!

✔ *Do* consider engaging a good health travel planner.

Even the most intrepid, adventurous medical traveler will benefit from the knowledge, experience, and in-country support these professionals can bring to any health journey. *Do* thoroughly research an agent before plunking down your deposit.

✔ *Do* get it in writing.

Cost estimates, appointments, recommendations, opinions, second opinions, airline and hotel arrangements—get as much as you can in writing, and *do* be sure to take all documentation with you on the plane. Email is fine, as long as you retain a written record of your key transactions. The more you get in writing, the less chance of a misunderstanding.

✔ *Do* insist on using a language you understand.

As much as many of us would like to have a better command of another language, the time to brush up on your Thai is most definitely *not* when negotiating medical care! Establishing comfortable, reliable communication with your key contacts is paramount to your success as a health traveler. Happily for English-speaking patients, most medical staff in Thailand's Joint Commission International (JCI)–accredited hospitals speak English, so communication should not be a problem.

✘ *Don't* plan your trip too tightly.

Don't plan your trip with military precision. A missed consultation or an extra two days of recovery in Thailand can mean expensive rescheduling with airlines. A good rule of thumb is to add an extra day for every five days you anticipate for consultation, treatment, and recovery.

✔ *Do* alert your bank and credit card companies.

Contact your bank and credit card companies *prior to your trip.* Inform them of your travel dates and where you will be. If you plan to use a credit card for large amounts, alert the company in advance, and reconfirm your credit limits to avoid card cancellation or unexpected rejections.

✔ *Do* learn a little about your destination.

Once you've decided on Thailand or any other health travel destination, spend a little time getting to know something about its history and geography. Buy or borrow a couple of travel guides. Read a local newspaper. Your hosts will appreciate your knowledge and interest.

✔ *Do* inform your local doctors before you leave.

Preserve a good working relationship with your family physician and local specialists. Although they may not particularly like your traveling overseas for medical care, most doctors will respect your decision. Your local healthcare providers need to know what you're doing, so they can continue your care and treatment once you return home.

WHILE IN THAILAND

✗ *Don't* be too adventurous with local cuisine.

One sure way to get your treatment off to a bad start is to enter your clinic with even a mild case of stomach upset due to a change in water or diet. Spicy Thai salads and *satays* are best sampled after your recovery. Thailand is famous for its hospitality, and Thai airlines, hotels, and hospitals will happily cater to your dietary needs. Prior to treatment, avoid rich, spicy foods and exotic drinks. Bottled water may be safest for your stomach. During any inpatient stay, *don't* be afraid to ask the hospital's dietician for a menu that's easy on your digestion. Hospitals, especially the ones listed here, have international patient coordinators who will help you order special meals, no matter what your tastes or dietary constraints.

✘ *Don't* scrimp on lodging.

Unless your finances absolutely demand it, avoid hotels and other accommodations in the "budget" category. You *don't* want to end up in uncomfortable surroundings when you're recuperating from major surgery. On the other hand, you should be able to find a good Thai hotel in a price range that suits you. Ask your hospital or health travel agent for a recommendation. You can find a wealth of hotel information at www.thaihotels.org.

✘ *Don't* stay too far from your treatment center.

When booking hotel accommodations for you and your companion, make sure the hospital or doctor's office is nearby. Staff members at your destination hospital can advise you on suitable lodging.

✘ *Don't* settle for second best in treatment options.

While you can cut corners on airfare, lodging, and transportation, always insist on the very best healthcare your money can buy. Focus on quality, not just price.

✔ *Do* befriend the staff.

Nurses, nurse's aides, paramedics, receptionists, clerks, and even maintenance people are vital members of your health team! Take the time to chat with them, learn their names, inquire about their families, and perhaps proffer a small gift. Above all, treat the staff with deference and respect. When you're ready to leave the hospital, a sincere thank-you note makes a great farewell.

GOING HOME

✘ *Don't* return home too soon.

After a long flight to Bangkok or Phuket, multiple consultations with physicians and staff, and a painful and disorienting medical procedure, you might feel ready to jump on the first flight home. That's understandable but not advisable. Your body needs time to recuperate, and your in-country physician needs to track your recovery progress. As you plan your trip, ask your physician how much recovery time is advised for your particular treatment— then add a few extra days, just to be safe. Thailand offers suitable options for rest and recovery, either close to your hospital or—if you are well enough—at a resort facility near Bangkok, Pattaya, or Hua Hin. Learn more at www.tourismthailand.org.

✔ *Do* set aside some of your medical travel savings for a vacation.

You and your companion deserve it! If you're not able to take leisure time during your trip to Thailand, then set aside a little money for some time off after you return home, even if it's only a weekend getaway.

✔ *Do* get all your paperwork before leaving the country.

Get copies of everything. No matter how eager you are to get well and get home, make sure you have full documentation on your procedure(s), treatment(s), and followup. Get receipts for everything.

ABOVE ALL, TRUST YOUR INTUITION

Your courage and good judgment have set you on the path to medical travel. Rely on your instincts. If, for example, you feel uncomfortable with your in-country consultation, switch doctors. If you get a queasy feeling about extra or uncharted costs, don't be afraid to question them. Thousands of health travelers have beaten a well-worn path abroad, using good information and common sense. You can, too! Safe travels!

Ten "Must-Ask" Questions for Your Candidate Physician

Make the following initial inquiries, either of your health travel agent or the physician(s) you're interviewing:

1. *What are your credentials? Where did you receive your medical degree? Where was your internship? What types of continuing education workshops have you attended recently?* The right international physician either has credentials posted on the Web or will be happy to email you a complete résumé.

2. *How many patients do you see each month?* Hopefully, it's more than 50 and less than 500. The physician who says "I don't know" should make you suspicious. Doctors should be in touch with their customer base and have such information readily available.

3. *To what associations do you belong?* Any worthwhile physician or surgeon is a member of at least one medical association. Your practitioner should be keeping good company with others in the field.

4. *How many patients have you treated who have had my condition?* There's safety in numbers, and you'll want to know them. Find out how many procedures your intended hospital has performed. Ask how many of *your specific treatments for your specific condition* your candidate doctor has personally conducted.

5. *What are the fees for your initial consultation?* Answers will vary, and you should compare prices to those of other physicians you interview.

6. *May I call you on your cell phone before, during, and after treatment?* Most international physicians stay in close, direct contact with their patients, and cell phones are their tools of choice.

7. *What medical and personal health records do you need to assess my condition and treatment needs?* Most physicians require at least the basics: recent notes and recommendations from consultations with your local physician or specialists, x-rays directly related to your condition, perhaps a medical history, and other health records. Be wary of the physician who requires no personal paperwork.

8. *Do you practice alone, or with others in a clinic or hospital?* Look for a physician who practices among a group of certified professionals with a broad range of related skills.

For surgery:

9. *Do you do the surgery yourself, or do you have assistants do the surgery?* This is one area where delegation isn't desirable. You want assurance that your procedure won't be performed by your practitioner's protégé.

10. *Are you the physician who oversees my entire treatment, including pre-surgery, surgery, prescriptions, physical therapy recommendations, and post-surgery checkups?* For larger surgical procedures, you want the designated team captain. While that's usually the surgeon, check to make sure.

CHAPTER TWO

Patients Beyond Borders
Budget Planner

As with any other trip, your health travel costs will depend largely upon your tastes, lifestyle preferences, length of stay, side trips, and pocketbook. A patient flying first-class and staying at a five-star hotel can naturally expect less of a savings than one who spends frequent-flyer miles and lodges in a modest—but perfectly satisfactory—three-star hotel.

To derive an estimate of your health travel costs and savings, we suggest you use the "*Patients Beyond Borders* Budget Planner" below. Don't feel pressured to fill in every line item in your Budget Planner. Focus on the big expenses first, such as treatment and airfare, and then fill in the remainder as your planning progresses. You probably won't use all the categories. For example, you may already have an up-to-date passport, or you may stay only at a hospital and never visit a hotel. The Budget Planner simply lists all the common health travel expenses. As you plan, fill in the blanks that apply to you, and you'll arrive at a rough estimate of your costs—and your savings. (You'll find more details in *Patients Beyond Borders: Second Edition.*)

A Few Notes on Costs

Passport and visa. US citizens who don't have a passport and are purchasing one for the first time should budget about $200 for fees, photographs, and shipping. Passport renewal in the US costs about $150. Passport and visa fees for other countries vary widely; check with the appropriate government office to determine Thailand's visa requirements. (See "The Medical Traveler's Essentials" in Part Four for details.)

Airfare. Air transportation will likely be your biggest non-treatment cost. It pays to shop hard for bargains. If you're okay flying coach, by all means do so; business- and first-class international travel are wildly expensive. If you have a *trusted* travel agency, use it, although with caution. Most have side deals with airlines, and their commissions and fees can cut into your savings. If you're comfortable using the Internet, take advantage of one of the many discount online travel agencies, such as Orbitz (www.orbitz.com), Expedia (www.expedia.com), Travelocity (www.travelocity.com), or CheapTickets (www.cheaptickets .com). Or go to individual airlines' Web sites, where you can sometimes snag special Internet fares.

International entry and exit fees. Many countries charge fees at the airport, and they may be due on arrival, on departure, or both. It's usually best to have cash in your pocket for these fees, which sometimes change dramatically without notice. At press time, Thailand was charging an airport tax of about US$21 for departing international passengers. That cost is usually included in the price of a prepaid air travel ticket.

Rental car. When traveling, some people feel they can't manage without a car. Yet international car rentals are expensive, big-city parking is a hassle, and driving in a foreign country can land you in the hospital well ahead of your scheduled stay. It's often better for the health traveler to use public transportation or taxis.

Mass transit. Bangkok's Airport Rail Link takes only 15 minutes to whisk travelers from the main international airport to Bangkok's central business district, and for a modest fare. If you're staying in Bangkok for a while, the Bangkok Transit System (BTS) Sky Train is a great way to get around; it's fast and cheap. In fact, it pays to stay at a hotel within walking distance of a Sky Train station. Fares can be purchased individually, but a BTS SmartPass is an inexpensive and convenient way to pay for multiple trips. For those adventurous or brave enough, motorcycle taxis go where the BTS doesn't, with fares normally less than 20 baht (about 60 US cents) for short distances. Bangkok also has an inexpensive Mass Rapid Transit (MRT) subway system.

Other transportation. Transportation to and from the airport in Thailand will probably be handled by the hospital, your health travel agent, or the hotel where you or your companion will reside. Budget for the cost of transportation to and from your airport back home, as well as for other transportation in Thailand. Taxis and buses are usually not expensive. Allow plenty of time, though, as Bangkok traffic can be heavy during rush hours, depending on the district. A budget allotment of US$100 should be more than adequate to cover your local transportation costs. (See Part Four for more details.)

Companions. Budget for the additional airfare and meals for your travel companion and—depending on whether you'll be doubling up—lodging. Items you can usually share include local taxi rides, mobile phone, and computer and Internet services. Items you can't share include passport and visa costs, airfare, airport fees and taxes, railway fares, meals, and entertainment.

Treatment. When you are evaluating a treatment center or physician, request the cost details in writing (email is okay), including the prices for basic treatment plus ancillaries, such as anesthesia, room fees, prescriptions, nursing services, and more. Other useful questions: Are meals included in my hospital stay? Do you supply a bed for my companion? Is there an Internet connection in the room or lobby? If you're using a health travel agency, make sure your representative gives you specific answers in writing to these important questions, along with a firm cost estimate for treatment and ancillary fees.

Lodging during treatment. These costs are straightforward and are largely a function of your tastes and pocketbook. Your doctor or your treatment center's staff can provide you with a list of preferred hotels nearby.

Post-treatment lodging. It's a good idea to stick around for at least a week post-treatment, because your physician will want to keep an eye on how your recovery is progressing. Many hospitals and clinics will help you arrange accommodations nearby and plan for nursing services to meet your post-treatment needs.

Meals. If you're staying in a hospital, most of your meals will probably be provided, and the food is often surprisingly good. Many hospitals offer reasonable meal plans for companions. Ask the facility or your agent about costs for hospital meals. Otherwise, budget your dining out according to taste, both for you and for your companion.

Tips. Tipping customs vary widely overseas. Tipping is not standard practice in Thailand, although that is beginning to change. If you do tip, it's best to do so in baht. Taxi drivers do not expect a tip, but the gesture is always appreciated. A tip of 20–50 baht is acceptable for porters. Larger hotels and restaurants add a 10 percent service charge to your bill.

Leisure travel. Many health travelers plan a vacation for either before or after treatment. Although this expense isn't strictly a part of your health travel budget, you may want to add the costs of vacation-related lodging, transportation, meals, and other expenses into your estimated budget.

The $6,000 Rule

A good monetary barometer of whether your medical trip is financially worthwhile is the *Patients Beyond Borders* "$6,000 Rule": If your total quote for local treatment (including consultations, procedures, and hospital stay) is US$6,000 or more, you'll probably save money by traveling abroad for your care. If it's less than US$6,000, you're likely better off having your treatment at home.

The application of this rule varies, of course, depending on your financial position and lifestyle preferences. For some, a small savings might offset the hassles of travel. For others who might be traveling anyway, savings considerations are fuzzier.

Will My Health Insurance Cover My Overseas Medical Expenses?

As of this writing, it's possible, but not probable. While the largest employers and healthcare insurers—not to mention ever-vocal politicians—struggle with new models of coverage, most plans do not yet cover the costs of obtaining treatment abroad. Yet, with healthcare costs threatening to literally bust some Western economies, pressures for change are mounting. Recognizing that the globalization of healthcare is now a reality—and that developed countries are falling behind—insurers, employers, and hospitals are beginning to form partnerships with payers and providers abroad. By the time you read this book, large insurers may already be offering coverage (albeit limited) across borders. Check with your insurer for the latest on your coverage abroad.

Can I Sue?

For better or worse, many countries do not share the Western attitude toward personal and institutional liability. A full discussion of the reasons lies outside the scope of this book. Here's a good rule of thumb: if legal recourse is a primary concern in making your health travel decision, you probably shouldn't head abroad for medical treatment.

If, however, you experience severe complications and do not receive the followup care you think you need or deserve, then you may want to consider legal action, say attorneys Amanda Hayes and Natasha Bellroth of Global MD. "Legal recourse and remedies are generally limited abroad for patients who experience bad outcomes in foreign facilities," they say. "Moreover, a patient's ability to sue a foreign physician or facility for medical malpractice is limited by the availability of an appropriate forum in which to bring a lawsuit."

For example, say Hayes and Bellroth, assume that American patient John Smith travels to Bangkok for hip replacement surgery at ABC Hospital and suffers a bad outcome caused by his surgeon's negligence. Mr. Smith has some options for pursuing a judicial remedy:

✦ In order to sue ABC Hospital in the US, a US court must be able to exercise jurisdiction over ABC Hospital, a corporation in Thailand with no offices or employees in the US. US courts may only assert general or specific personal jurisdiction over a foreign entity when the foreign entity's presence or dealings where the suit is brought justify requiring the company to defend the suit there.

✦ Assuming that the case proceeds in the US to judgment against ABC Hospital, Mr. Smith faces an uphill battle to enforce an American judgment in Thailand. If Mr. Smith wins a large punitive damages award from an American court, he will be disappointed to learn that punitive damages are rarely awarded outside of the US and are unlikely to be enforced (in any of the countries currently attracting American medical travelers).

✦ Alternatively, Mr. Smith may try to sue ABC Hospital in Bangkok, which requires that he hire a lawyer in Thailand and perhaps travel back to Thailand to attend the proceedings. Even if Mr. Smith prevails in the suit, he will probably only be able to recover his actual damages (the provable out-of-pocket cost of harm caused by negligence, e.g., medical bills incurred for corrective surgery and lost wages due to time away from work), as few countries award punitive damages to successful plaintiffs.

✦ Mr. Smith may seek to arbitrate his claim against ABC Hospital before an international tribunal. For example, the International Court of Arbitration of the International Chamber of Commerce may provide Mr. Smith with a viable and likely more cost-effective way to hold ABC Hospital accountable for negligence. Generally, an agreement to arbitrate claims must have been in place before the relationship commenced. Mr. Smith should have confirmed that prior to surgery, ABC Hospital had agreed to arbitration of potential future claims and to where those proceedings would occur.

Each alternative forum presents its own unique set of challenges. There is no ideal solution that would put judicial recourse against a foreign entity on par with the remedies available against a US hospital or physician. There are, however, practical measures that Mr. Smith might have taken before he traveled to Thailand that would have helped him manage the risk in the unlikely event of a bad outcome:

✦ For example, Mr. Smith might have purchased insurance (a health travel agency should be able to point the patient to available policies) designed specifically to protect him from the financial consequences of foreseeable complications and unforeseeable medical malpractice. Such insurance could have helped Mr. Smith eliminate the cost of legal action while compensating him up to the amount of the policy limit he purchased.

✦ In addition, had Mr. Smith paid for his procedure with a major credit card, his card company may have allowed him to recover the cost of a disappointing treatment by disputing the charges.

✦ Finally, Mr. Smith could have made sure that his health travel agency and the treating facility had a clear and reasonable protocol in place for dealing with bad outcomes and complications. Ideally, the hospital would have agreed to absorb costs associated with making Mr. Smith whole again (return flight, accommodations, and corrective procedure) and to compensate him if he could be satisfied.

Ultimately, there is no perfect way to compensate a patient (either domestically or abroad) who has suffered an imperfect outcome after a medical procedure. The good news is that informed patients can take preventive measures to protect themselves before they travel abroad for care, so they do not end up in the hands of imperfect healthcare insurance and judicial systems.

Furthermore, foreign hospitals are eager to prove that the quality of their surgeons and technical facilities rivals or even exceeds that found in Western nations. Your independent research will reveal that sophisticated foreign hospitals and governments are heavily invested in serving international patients with high-quality healthcare; they understand that the publicity associated with even one bad outcome could quickly end the growing flow of health travelers.

Patients Beyond Borders Budget Planner

Item	Cost	Comment
IN-COUNTRY		
Passport/Visa	$200.00	For passport and visa, non-expedited
Rush charges, if any:		
Treatment Estimate		
Procedure:		
Hospital room, if extra:		Often included in treatment package
Lab work, x-rays, etc.:		
Additional consultations:		
Tips/gifts for staff:	$100.00	
Other:		
Other:		
Post-Treatment		
Recuperation lodging:		Hospital room or hotel
Physical therapy:		
Prescriptions:		
Concierge services:		Optional
Other:		
Other:		
Airfare		
You:		
Your companion:		
Other travelers:		
Airport fees:		
Other:		
Other:		
In-Country Transportation		
Taxis, buses, limos:	$200.00	
Rental car:		
Other:		
Other:		

(continued)

Patients Beyond Borders Budget Planner (*continued*)

Item	Cost	Comment
Room and Board		
Hotel:		
Food:		
Entertainment/sightseeing:		
Other:		
Other:		
"While You're Away" Costs		
Pet sitter/house sitter:		
Other:		
Other:		
IN-COUNTRY SUBTOTAL		
HOMETOWN		
Procedure:		
Lab work, x-rays, etc.:		
Hospital room, if extra:		
Additional consultations:		
Physical therapy:		
Prescriptions:		
Other:		
Other:		
HOMETOWN SUBTOTAL		
TOTAL SAVINGS:		Subtract In-Country Subtotal
		from Hometown Subtotal

Patients Beyond Borders Sample Budget Planner

Item	Cost	Comment
IN-COUNTRY		
Passport/Visa	$200.00	For passport and visa, non-expedited
Rush charges, if any:		
Treatment Estimate		
Procedure:	$9,000.00	
Hospital room, if extra:		Often included in treatment package
Lab work, x-rays, etc.:	$45.00	
Additional consultations:	$200.00	
Tips/gifts for staff:	$100.00	
Other:		
Other:		
Post-Treatment		
Recuperation lodging:	$1,100.00	Hospital room or hotel
Physical therapy:	$65.00	
Prescriptions:	$65.00	
Concierge services:	$300.00	Optional
Other:		
Other:		
Airfare		
You:	$880.00	
Your companion:	$880.00	
Other travelers:		
Airport fees:	$12.00	
Other:		
Other:		
In-Country Transportation		
Taxis, buses, limos:	$200.00	
Rental car:		
Other:		
Other:		

(continued)

Patients Beyond Borders Sample Budget Planner (*continued*)

Item	Cost	Comment
Room and Board		
Hotel:	$1,500.00	
Food:	$650.00	
Entertainment/sightseeing:	$500.00	
Other:		
Other:		
"While You're Away" Costs		
Pet sitter/house sitter:	$300.00	
Other:		
Other:		
IN-COUNTRY SUBTOTAL	$15,997.00	
HOMETOWN		
Procedure:	$55,000.00	
Lab work, x-rays, etc.:	$375.00	
Hospital room, if extra:	$4,400.00	
Additional consultations:	$1,200.00	
Physical therapy:	$400.00	
Prescriptions:	$500.00	
Other:		
Other:		
HOMETOWN SUBTOTAL	$61,875.00	
TOTAL SAVINGS:	$45,878.00	Subtract In-Country Subtotal
		from Hometown Subtotal

Your Medical Trip May Be Tax-Deductible

What do *satays*, taxi rides, and treatments have in common? Depending on the country you live in, these expenses may be tax-deductible as part of your health travel. In the US, for example, depending upon your income level and cost of treatment, some or most of your health journey can be itemized as a straight deduction from your adjusted gross income.

In brief, if you're itemizing your deductions in the US, and if qualifying medical treatment and related expenses amount to more than 7.5 percent of adjusted gross income, the Internal Revenue Service allows US citizens to deduct the remainder of those expenses, whether they were incurred in Toledo, Ohio, or Toledo, Spain.

For example, if a US citizen's adjusted gross income is US$90,000, then any allowed medical expense over $6,750 ($90,000 x 7.5 percent) becomes a straight deduction. Suppose that a medical trip costs a total of $14,000, including treatment, travel, lodging, and, of course, a two-week surgeon-recommended stay in a five-star beachfront recuperation resort; for that trip, the deduction from the US medical traveler's adjusted gross income could be $7,250 ($14,000 minus $6,750).

Of course, the expenses must be directly related to the treatment, and many specific items are disallowed. Examples of typical tax-deductible items include

- any treatment normally covered by a health insurance plan
- transportation expenses, including air, train, boat, or road travel
- lodging and in-treatment meals
- recovery hotels, surgical retreats, and recuperation resorts

Medical travelers should save all receipts and keep a detailed expense log, noting time, date, purpose, and amount paid. If you are planning to take a tax deduction, ask for letters and other documentation from your in-country healthcare provider, particularly any recommendations made for outside lodging, special diets, and other services.

For more information, US citizens can go to www.irs.gov or call 800 829.1040. Medical travelers from other countries should check their government's tax policies. It's always a good idea to consult a competent tax advisor with questions or concerns.

CHAPTER THREE

Checklists
for Health Travel

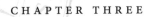

If you're like most readers of this book, you're *almost* sure that health travel is the right choice. You have a diagnosis and you know what medical procedure is required. You've reviewed the costs for your procedure at home and are beginning to believe that treatment abroad offers significant advantages—mostly financial.

But, if you're like most patients contemplating medical travel, you know you have some homework to do before you get on a plane and head to a hospital or clinic abroad. While this book focuses primarily on destinations for treatment in Thailand, it's a good idea to reconsider some of the questions that apply to all health travelers, no matter what their treatment or destination.

The seven checklists that follow will remind you of some important issues and items. Review and check off those things that apply to your situation, and you'll increase your chances of a safe, happy, and healthy outcome. If you desire additional information about traveling abroad for treatment, you may want to buy or borrow a copy of *Patients Beyond Borders: Second Edition,* which contains greatly expanded information for medical travelers.

CHECKLIST 1: *Should I Consult a Health Travel Planner?*

Health travel planners answer to many names: brokers, facilitators, agents, expeditors. Throughout this book, we use the phrase "health travel planner" or "health travel agent" to mean any agency or representative who specializes in helping patients obtain medical treatment abroad. (Several agencies are profiled in Part Two.) Before engaging the services of a health travel agent, ask yourself these questions:

WHETHER TO USE A HEALTH TRAVEL PLANNER	Yes	No	Not Sure	Notes to Myself
Will a health travel planner save me time?				
Am I willing to pay for the convenience of a health travel planner's services?				
Will I feel more confident about health travel if I use the services of an agency?				
Does the agent I'm considering have the knowledge and experience I need?				
Does this planner have a track record of successful service to the health traveler?				
Does this agent speak my language well enough for us to converse comfortably?				
Can I get at least two recommendations or letters of reference from former clients of this agency? Have I checked these references?				
Can I get at least two recommendations or letters of reference from treatment centers that work with this agency? Have I checked these references?				
Can this agency give me complete information about possible destinations and options for my procedure?				

(continued)

WHETHER TO USE A HEALTH TRAVEL PLANNER	Yes	No	Not Sure	Notes to Myself
Will this agent put me in touch with one or more treatment centers and physicians?				
Will this agent work collaboratively to help me choose the best treatment option?				
Is this agent responsive to my questions and concerns?				
Does the service package this agent is offering meet my needs?				
Does this agent have longstanding affiliations with in-country treatment centers and practitioners?				
Has this planner negotiated better-than-retail rates with hospitals, clinics, physicians, hotels, and (perhaps) airlines?				
Can this agent save me money on other in-country costs, such as airport pickup and dropoff or transportation to my clinic?				
Can this agent provide personal assistance and support in my destination country?				
Is this planner willing to work within the constraints of my budget?				
Do I know (and have in writing) the exact costs for this agency's services?				
Do I have a suitable contract or letter of agreement with this agency?				
Do I feel comfortable with this agency? Have we built a sense of trust?				

When *Not* to Use a Health Travel Planner

Don't use an agent who does not promptly answer your initial requests for information, does not reasonably follow through on commitments, or does not treat you well in any way. Difficulty deciphering an agent's communications is a red flag, too. If a trusted friend or other reliable source has referred you to a specific clinic and physician, then half the work is already done, and you may want to forgo an agent's services, particularly if the hospital or clinic provides similar services (for instance, through its international patients center).

Paying for a Health Travel Planner's Services

Some planners offer "all-in-one" package deals, which are fine. However, at tax time, you may need to show your itemized cost breakdown, including treatment, lodging, meals, transportation, and health travel agent fees. Spreadsheets are universal these days. Ask your planner to give you a detailed expense log.

Costs and payments are usually handled in one of three ways:

- **Membership, upfront fee required.** This arrangement requires the patient to pay a nonrefundable membership fee (often in the US$50 – 300 range) before any services are rendered. The membership fee is usually folded into the package price if you engage that agent.

- **Package, advance deposit required.** In this arrangement, an agent first provides enough information to get you well along your path: data on specific treatment centers and physicians, advice on medical records and in-country procedures, and perhaps even a telephone consultation with your candidate physician or surgeon. At that point, if you decide to engage the agent, you'll be asked to submit a deposit, perhaps 25–50 percent of the entire package price. Another payment is due prior to treatment, and the remainder is payable when you leave the hospital or clinic.

- **Pay as you go, direct to third parties.** A handful of planners act more as referral services than as full-blown brokers, providing information about hospitals and physicians, airfares, and vacation opportunities, without doing much of the real legwork. They usually charge you a commission or set fee on any service you engage.

If you're dealing with a reputable agent, all these fee structures get you to much the same place. Beware, however, of agents asking for 100 percent up front. You should see evidence of performance, communicate with all the parties personally (via telephone or email), and know that your hard-earned money is going where it should.

Although a deposit of up to 50 percent of the total package cost is usually required, you should reserve at least 25 percent of the total bill for final payment. In other words, as with most other services, don't pay the entire bill until you're satisfied and all the services you were promised have been provided. Most planners accept credit cards, but before you use yours, ask your agent about any surcharges associated with credit card payments.

CHECKLIST 2: *How Can a Health Travel Planner Help Me?*

Of all the services a health travel planner offers, the most important are related to your treatment. Start your dialogue by asking the fundamental questions: Do you know the best doctors? Have you met personally with your preferred physicians and visited their clinics? Can you give me their credentials and background information? What about accommodations? Do you provide transportation to and from the airport? To and from the treatment center? If an agent is knowledgeable and capable with these details, the rest of the planning usually takes care of itself.

DOES MY HEALTH TRAVEL PLANNER PROVIDE THIS SERVICE?	Yes	No	Not Sure	Notes to Myself
Treatment options from which to choose destination countries, hospitals, and physicians best equipped to meet my needs				
Information on hospital accreditation and physicians' credentials, board affiliations, number of surgeries performed, association memberships, and ongoing training				
Appointment scheduling and confirmations for tests, consultations, and treatments				
Teleconsultation with physicians or surgeons to review my medical history and discuss my procedure				
Transfer of medical records, including history, x-rays/scans, test results, recommendations, and other documentation				
Travel arrangements, including airline and hotel reservations, tickets, and confirmations; also including local in-country transportation				
Visa or passport facilitation				
Onsite pre-treatment assistance, including a local representative to accompany me to appointments, expedite hospital admission, arrange local transportation, and assist with my hospital discharge				
Recovery arrangements, including local transportation, lodging, meals, and any nursing services required during recovery				

(continued)

DOES MY HEALTH TRAVEL PLANNER PROVIDE THIS SERVICE?	Yes	No	Not Sure	Notes to Myself
Amenity arrangements, including "concierge services," such as take-out food from restaurants, tickets for events, and dry-cleaning and laundry services				
Communications arrangements, including telephone, cell phone, and Internet services				
Leisure or vacation planning (if desired)				
Aftercare and followup once I've returned home, including post-treatment liaison for information retrieval and making arrangements for a return trip should complications arise				

CHECKLIST 3: *What Do I Need to Do Ahead of Time?*

Although each journey varies according to the traveler's preferences and pocketbook, good planning is essential to the success of any trip. That goes double for the medical traveler. This checklist covers some of the planning you'll need to do to become a fully prepared and informed global patient.

Why should you plan at least three months in advance?

- **The best physicians are also the busiest.** If you want the most qualified physician and the best care your global patient money can buy, give the doctors and treatment centers you select plenty of time to work you into their calendars.

- **The lowest international airfares go to those who book early.** Booking at least 60 days prior to treatment avoids the unhappy upward spiral of air travel costs. If you're planning to redeem frequent-flyer miles, try to book at least 90 days in advance.

- **Peak seasons can snarl the best-laid plans.** International tourism attracts large numbers of people, and you can encounter problems if you want or need to travel during the busy tourist season.

- **Everything takes longer than you think it will.** It's simply a fact of life.

For Big Surgeries, Think Big

You want to be certain you're getting the best. For big surgeries, I advise heading to the big hospitals that have performed large numbers of *exactly* your kind of procedure, with the accreditation and success ratios to prove it. A hospital accredited by the Joint Commission International (JCI)—such as Samitivej Sukhumvit Hospital in Bangkok—carries the necessary staff, medical talent, administrative infrastructure, state-of-the-art instrumentation, and institutional followup you need. (**Note:** For more information on accreditation, see "The What and Why of JCI" and "Alternatives to JCI" below.)

Be sure to ask about the success and morbidity rates *for your particular procedure* and find out how they compare with those at home. If you are having surgery, ask your surgeon how many surgeries *of exactly your procedure* he or she has performed in the past two years. While there are no set standards, fewer than ten is not so good. More than 50 is much better.

HAVE I COMPLETED THESE PLANNING STEPS?	Yes	No	Notes to Myself
Engaged the services of a health travel planner (if desired — see Checklists 1 and 2)			
Obtained a second opinion — or a third if necessary — on diagnosis and treatment options			
Considered a range of treatment options and discussed each option with potential providers			
Reviewed the various hospitals, clinics, specialties, and treatments available to select an appropriate destination (see Part Two)			
Chosen a reliable, fun travel companion			
Obtained and reviewed the professional credentials of two or more physicians or surgeons (see "Ten 'Must-Ask' Questions for Your Candidate Physician" in Chapter One)			
Selected the best physician or surgeon for the treatment I need			
Researched the history and accreditation of the hospital or clinic (see "The What and Why of JCI" and "Alternatives to JCI" below)			
Checked for the affiliations and partnerships of the hospital or clinic			
Learned about the number of surgeries performed in the hospital or clinic (generally, the more the better)			
Learned about success rates (these are usually calculated as a ratio of successful operations to the overall number of operations performed)			
Gathered and sent all medical records and diagnostic information that my physician or surgeon needs to plan my treatment			
Prearranged travel, accommodations, recovery, and leisure activities (if desired)			
Prearranged amenities, such as concierge services in-country or wheelchair services on the return trip			
Packed the essentials (see Checklist 4)			
Double-checked everything — then checked again			

The What and Why of JCI

When you walk into a hospital or clinic in the US and many other Western countries, chances are good that it's accredited, meaning that it's in compliance with standards and "good practices" set by an independent accreditation agency. In the US, by far the largest and most respected accreditation agency is the Joint Commission. The commission casts a wide net of evaluation for hospitals, clinics, home healthcare, ambulatory services, and a host of other healthcare facilities and services throughout the US.

Responding to a global demand for accreditation standards, in 1999 the Joint Commission launched JCI, its international affiliate accreditation agency. In order to be accredited, an international healthcare provider must meet the rigorous standards set forth by JCI. At this writing, some 240 hospitals, laboratories, and special programs outside the US have been JCI-approved, with more coming on board each month.

Although JCI accreditation is not essential, it's an important new benchmark and the only medically oriented seal of approval for international hospitals and clinics. Learning that your treatment center is JCI-approved lends a comfort to the process, and the remainder of your searching and checking need not be as rigorous. That said, many excellent hospitals, while not JCI-approved, have received local accreditation at the same levels as the world's best treatment centers.

JCI's Web site carries far more information than you'll ever want to explore on accreditation standards and procedures. To view JCI's current roster of accredited hospitals abroad, go to www.joint commissioninternational.org/JCI-Accredited-Organizations.

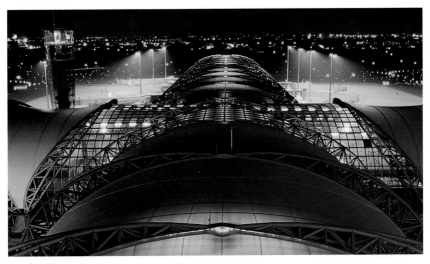

Bangkok's new Suvarnabhumi International Airport

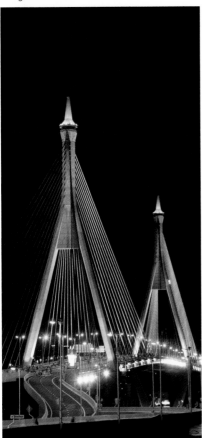

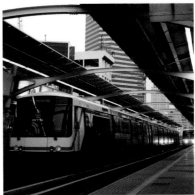

The Sky Train helps beat Bangkok traffic

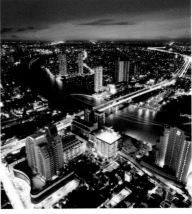

The Mega Bridge in Bangkok

Night view of the Chao Phraya River

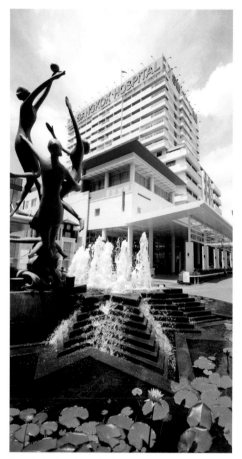

Bangkok Hospital exterior

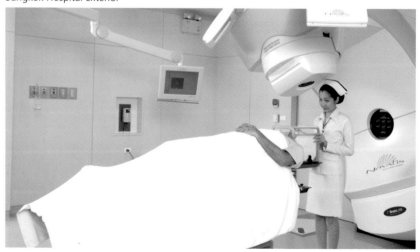

Live music in the lobby

Bangkok Hospital sets new standards in patient care.

State-of-the-art instrumentation throughout the facility

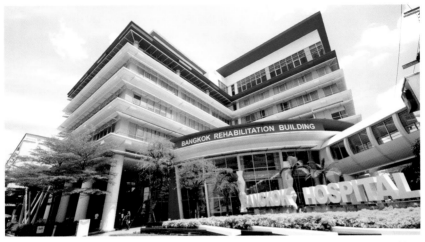

Bangkok Hospital Rehabilitation Building

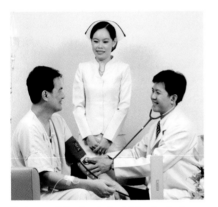

Patient satisfaction is the highest priority

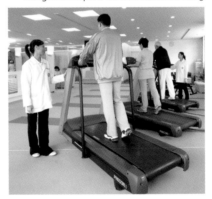

Physical Therapy Unit

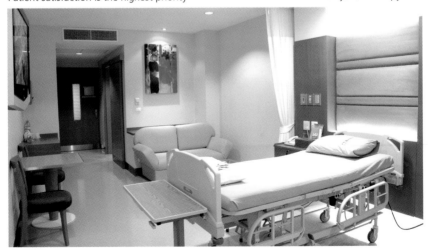

Spacious single-bed patient room

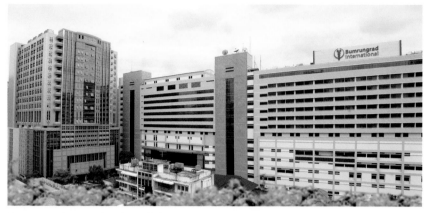

Bumrungrad International Hospital

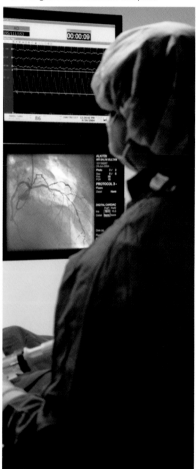

Cardiac imaging for diagnosis and
evaluation

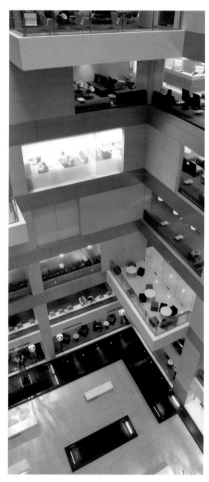

Bumrungrad's beautiful new 22-floor
outpatient clinic

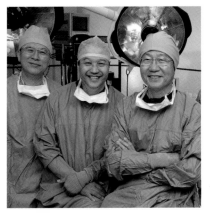
Internationally trained physicians

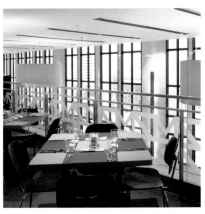
World-class dining

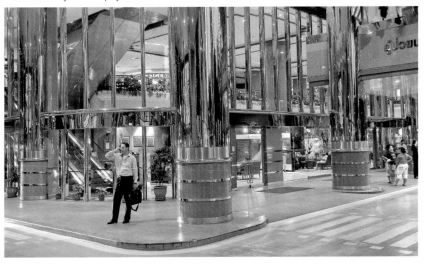
Bumrungrad's entrance and valet parking

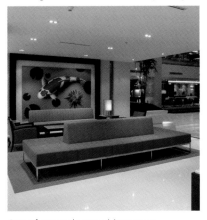
One of many elegant visitor areas

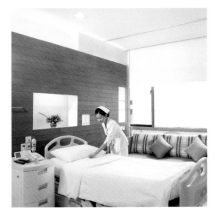
Single-bed patient room

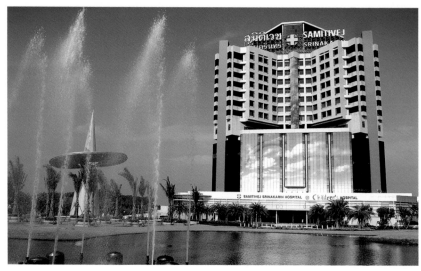

Samitivej Srinakarin Hospital

Samitivej
Hospitals offer
high-quality
medical services
and modern
technology.

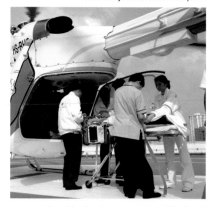

Samitivej's air transport and helipad

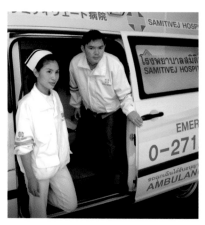

24/7 ambulatory transport

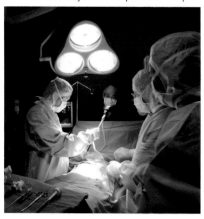

One of Samitivej's many operating theaters

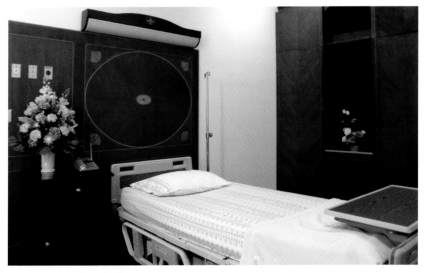

Samitivej's presidential suite

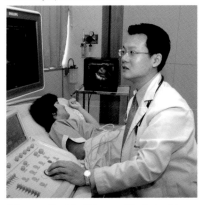

JCI-accredited facilities, certified physicians

Samitivej Srinakarin Hospital provides superior care and comprehensive medical services.

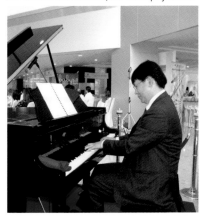

Pianist in Samitivej's friendly lobby

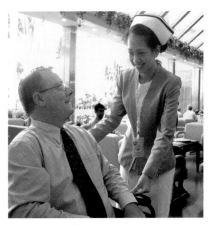

Caring staff tend to patients' every need

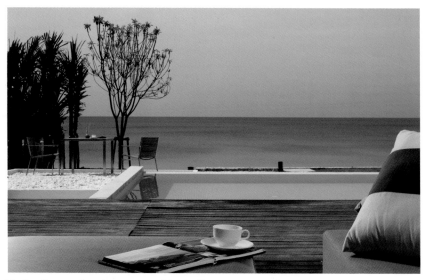

Thailand's many beach resorts provide excellent recovery options

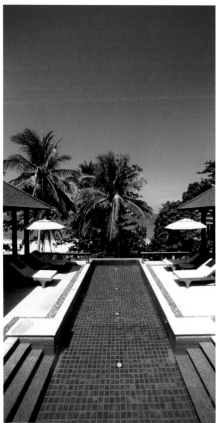

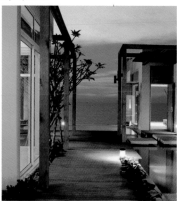

Peaceful recuperation and wellness

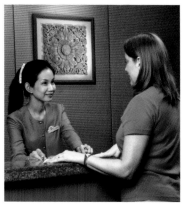

Coastal villa resort

Friendly service in "the Land of Smiles"

Alternatives to JCI

When researching hospitals and clinics abroad, you'll often come across the phrase "ISO-accredited." Based in Geneva, Switzerland, the International Organization for Standardization (ISO) is a 157-country network of national standards institutes that approves and accredits a wide range of product and service sectors worldwide, including hospitals and clinics. ISO mostly oversees facilities and administration, not healthcare procedures, practices, or methods.

Other organizations in other countries set standards and accredit hospitals. Organizations that accredit in non-JCI countries include the International Society for Quality in Healthcare, the Australian Council of Healthcare Standards, the Canadian Council on Health Services Accreditation, the Council for Health Services Accreditation of Southern Africa, the Egyptian Health Care Accreditation Organization, the Irish Health Services Accreditation Board, the Japan Council for Quality Health Care, and many more. If you are considering a hospital accredited by any organization, it's wise to investigate the criteria applied to the accreditation and determine to your own satisfaction that the standards are sufficient and appropriate to your needs.

CHECKLIST 4: *What Should I Pack?*

You've likely heard the cardinal rule of international travel: pack light. Less to carry means less to lose. Don't worry if you leave behind some basic item, such as shampoo or a comb; you can always pick it up at your destination. That said, this checklist covers the items you absolutely, positively shouldn't forget—and make sure you carry these things in your carry-on bag. A prescription or passport lost in checked luggage could spell disaster.

IS THIS ITEM PACKED IN MY CARRY-ON BAG?	Yes	No	Notes to Myself
Passport			
Visa (if required)			
Travel itinerary			
Airline tickets or eticket confirmations			
Driver's license or valid picture ID (in addition to passport)			
Health insurance card(s) or policy			
ATM card or traveler's checks			
Credit card(s)			
Enough cash for airport fees and local transportation on arrival			
Immunization record			
Prescription medications			
Hard-to-find over-the-counter drugs			
Medical records, current x-rays/scans, consultations, and treatment notes			
All financial agreements and hard copies of email correspondence			
Phone and fax numbers, mailing addresses, and email addresses of people I need or want to contact in-country			
Phone and fax numbers, mailing addresses, and email addresses of people I need or want to contact back home			
Travel journal for notes, expense records, and receipts			

CHECKLIST 5: *What Should I Do Just Before and During My Trip?*

Now that you've made appointments with one or more physicians, booked your flights and hotel, and arranged transportation, the hard part is behind you—except, of course, for the treatment itself. You'll find that once you arrive in Thailand, you will be greeted graciously with help and support from hotel and hospital staff, your health travel agent, and sometimes even a friendly bystander.

If you haven't done much international traveling prior to this health journey, keep in mind that you don't need to be a seasoned travel veteran to have a successful trip. Getting things done cooperatively and efficiently will help you and your companion preserve your physical *and* mental health. Knowing a little something about the culture, history, geography, and language of your host country will buy you boatloads of goodwill and appreciation. (The information in Part Four of this book will get you off to a good start.)

Tick off the items on this checklist to make sure you stay safe, happy, and well before and during your trip.

PREPARATIONS FOR MY TRIP	Yes	No	Not Sure	Notes to Myself
Have I read (or at least skimmed) a travel book or some brochures about the history, culture, and government of my destination country?				
Have I learned a few phrases, such as "please" and "thank you," in the local language?				
Have I studied a map of the city or country?				
Do I know what the local currency is, what the exchange rate is, and how I can pay for my needs in my destination country?				
Do I know the rules about the amount of cash I can carry into and out of my destination country?				
Have I found out what extra fees I will be charged for using my credit cards or ATM cards abroad?				
If I want to use traveler's checks, am I sure that my service providers will accept them? (Some don't.)				

(continued)

PREPARATIONS FOR MY TRIP	Yes	No	Not Sure	Notes to Myself
Am I leaving my valuables at home?				
If I must carry valuables, am I sure that a hotel safe or a safe-deposit box will be available to me?				
Am I prepared to drink only bottled water and eat only cooked foods? (This is a wise precaution for both the health traveler and the companion.)				
Have I packed a sanitizer for cleaning my hands everywhere I travel?				
Have I packed comfortable clothes that are sensitive to local customs of dress?				
Have I made arrangements for telephone and email services that will allow me to stay in touch with friends and relatives back home? With service providers in-country?				
Am I sure my cell phone will work in-country?				
Have I informed my doctor of all my pre-existing health conditions, such as diabetes, heart disease, ulcers, and others?				
Have I informed my physician about all prescription and over-the-counter drugs I am taking, including vitamins, minerals, and herbal supplements?				
Am I following my doctor's instructions pre-treatment, such as going off certain drugs, losing weight, or avoiding alcohol?				

Continuity of Care—Critical to Success

Continuity of care can be a challenge for patients who travel for medical procedures, say Steven Gerst, MD, and John Linss of MedicaView International (www.medicaview.com). Typically, the patient's primary physician diagnoses the condition and then suggests treatment. But when the patient chooses to travel to another location or country to receive the treatment, the primary physician is too often left out of the process.

Similarly—and amazingly—many traveling patients engage a facility to perform a procedure without speaking directly to the surgeon before arriving. The patient and the hospital's international patient services coordinator may use email for preliminary communications. There may also be a telephone call or two with the coordinator. But the surgeon may not become actively involved until the patient arrives at the facility.

Too many patients make the assumption that a diagnosis is "the end of the story" and that contact with the coordinator is all that is required. *They could not be more wrong!*

Establish Communication!

Insist on speaking to the surgeon who will perform the procedure *before* you schedule your travel. You may communicate via teleconference, videoconference, or voice over Internet protocol (VOIP).

It is equally important that you establish communication between your primary (local) doctor and your in-country surgeon, so followup care will be prearranged. Because of time zone and language differences, this advance planning may be difficult, but it is essential. Complications and misunderstandings can arise if your doctors are not communicating properly. For example, after a knee replacement or a kidney transplant, many concerns and complications can arise during the long recuperation period. Lack of communication can result in unnecessary hardships and potential returns to surgery.

Once you choose to go outside your physician's primary network, few mechanisms currently exist to encourage and facilitate ongoing consultations. *You must establish your own.* Critical information about your case can be lost if you don't. *Be proactive!* Here and abroad, it is usually up to you to keep the dialogue going between your physicians.

Persistence is important, and the time-delayed effectiveness of email comes in handy—once you get the doctors in the habit of emailing each other and you. A secure online collaboration tool is even better, because it can keep all communications in one place and available to all participants at any time.

Have Your Most Current Medical Records

Once you have established contact with a doctor (or surgeon) and facility abroad, provide them with your most current medical records. If you have a chronic condition and you've finally said "enough," your medical records may be a year or more old. If they are, visit your local physician to obtain new laboratory tests, x-rays, or scans—whatever your in-country provider needs.

Medical records can be transmitted in two ways: you can send paper copies or disks by postal service, or you can send electronic documents via a secure online service. An online service is preferable for several reasons. First, it gets the records in the hands of the surgeon more quickly. Second, it creates a secure repository that can be accessed by both your local and overseas doctors. Third and most importantly, digital records create a foundation for aftercare collaboration.

Collaboration Between Your Local Doctor and Your Doctor Abroad

Transferring your medical records may get your local doctor communicating with your in-country doctor for the first time. This communication can be achieved though email, telephone, or a private group set-up in an online environment specifically designed for that purpose. Often such an environment is part of an online repository system that provides a secure place for collaboration between the doctors via protected blog, chat, email, and VOIP. Ask your doctor or health planner if such a system is available for your destination.

The next collaboration between doctors should occur after surgery. The surgeon should notify your local physician, preferably through an online system, of the details of the surgery and the aftercare protocol.

Once you return home and are again under the care of your local physician, this collaboration and consultation should continue until you are released from care with a clean bill of health.

Complete Documentation

Frequently, when such a repository system is not utilized, patients return home lacking the complete documentation their local physician needs to oversee ongoing care. The absence of information compromises the physician's effectiveness and threatens the patient's health.

Be sure to ask the surgical facility if access is available to an electronic system of medical record-sharing and physician collaboration. If not, request that your healthcare providers abroad subscribe to one to ensure that you can keep your local physician informed.

At a minimum, make sure your in-country facility provides you with complete records when you return home. Also make sure to keep your local physician involved from the first day. Good continuity of care is essential for a successful outcome.

Remember, as a patient, you need to take responsibility for the quality and consistency of the care you receive. If you don't, no one else will!

CHECKLIST 6: *What Do I Do After My Procedure?*

You've been out of surgery for two days, you hurt all over, your digestive system is acting up, and you're running a fever. Have you somehow contracted an antibiotic-resistant staph infection? Coping with post-surgery discomfort is difficult enough when you're close to home. Lying for long hours in a hospital bed, far away from family—that's often the darkest time for a health traveler.

Knowledge is the best antidote to needless worry. As with pre-surgery preparation, ask lots of questions about post-surgery discomforts *before* heading into the operating room. Be sure to ask doctors and nurses about what kinds of discomforts to expect following your specific procedure.

If your discomfort or pain becomes acute, bleeding is persistent, or you suspect a growing infection, you may be experiencing a complication that is more serious than mere discomfort and requires immediate attention. Contact your physician without delay.

This checklist will help you make the most of your post-treatment period and know when it's appropriate to seek medical assistance.

POST-PROCEDURE PREPARATIONS AND FOLLOWUP	Yes	No	Not Sure	Notes to Myself
Have I received all my doctor's instructions for my post-treatment care and recovery? Do I understand them all?				
Am I following all of my physician's instructions *to the letter*?				
Do I know what post-treatment signs and symptoms are normal?				
Do I know what post-treatment signs and symptoms indicate a need for prompt medical attention? (See "Post-Treatment: Normal Discomfort or Something More Complicated?" below.)				
Do I have copies of all my medical records and treatment records, including x-rays/scans, photographs, blood test results, prescriptions, and others?				
Do I have itemized receipts for all the bills I have paid?				
Do I have itemized bills for all the costs I have not yet paid?				
Do I have completed insurance claim forms (if applicable)?				
Have I allotted ample time for recovery?				
Do I know how to prevent blood clots in the legs after surgery and on the airplane? (See "Caution: Blood Clots in the Veins" below.)				
Do I know what followup treatment I will need when I return home, including physical therapy?				
Have I let my family know what help I will need when I return home?				
Have I checked in with my local doctor to share information about the procedure I had and my post-treatment care needs?				
Am I staying mentally, physically, and socially active following my procedure?				

Post-Treatment: Normal Discomfort or Something More Complicated?

Prior to your surgery, your doctor should thoroughly explain the procedure and tell you about discomforts you can expect after being wheeled out of the operating unit. Discomforts differ from complications. Discomforts are predictable and unthreatening. Complications, while rarely life threatening, are more serious and may require medical attention. These are some common discomforts you can expect following surgery:

✦ minor local pain and general achiness

✦ swelling

✦ puffiness

✦ bruising, swelling, and minor bleeding around the incision

✦ headaches (side effect of anesthesia)

✦ urinary retention or difficulty urinating (side effect of anesthesia and catheters)

✦ nausea and vomiting, dry mouth, temporary memory loss, lingering tiredness (all common side effects of anesthesia)

✦ hunger and undernutrition

Most surgically induced discomforts recede or disappear altogether during the first few days after treatment, as the body and spirit return to normal. Be sure, however, to report discomforts that persist or become more pronounced, as they might be early warning signs of more serious complications.

Complications vary according to each surgery, and you should make sure you're aware of the more common ones. Complications are scary, and many doctors would rather not go into morbid detail about them unless pressed. Complications are rare; most arise in less than 5 percent of all cases—and generally among patients who are aged or infirm in the first place. So while it's wise to be informed and vigilant, there's no need to worry yourself sick anticipating the worst. Common symptoms of complications include the following:

✦ infection, increased pain, or swelling around the incision

✦ abnormal bleeding around the incision

✦ sudden or unexplained high fever

✦ extreme chest pain or shortness of breath

✦ extreme headache

✦ extreme difficulty urinating

If you experience any of those symptoms, call your physician immediately.

Caution: Blood Clots in the Veins

Recent surgery and the immobility of long flights increase the risk of deep vein thrombosis (DVT), which is the formation of a clot, or thrombus, in one of the deep veins, usually in the lower leg. The symptoms of DVT may include pain and redness of the skin over a vein, or swelling and tenderness in the ankle, foot, or thigh. More serious symptoms include chest pain and shortness of breath.

You can take preventive steps to reduce your risk of DVT, such as wearing compression stockings and moving about frequently when on planes and trains. Ask your doctor about how soon after surgery you can safely undertake a long, sedentary trip.

OTHER WAYS TO REDUCE DVT RISKS

Before you travel:

- Stop smoking.
- Lose weight if you need to.
- Get enough exercise to be at least minimally fit before your surgery and your travel.
- Discuss stopping birth control pills and hormone replacement therapy with your doctor.
- Travel on an airline that provides sufficient leg room.
- Wear loose clothing.
- Reserve an aisle seat on the airplane so you can get up and move around easily.
- Ask your surgeon about using a pneumatic compression device during and after surgery.
- Before your flight home, ask your surgeon if you need an anticoagulant.
- Walk briskly for at least half an hour before takeoff.

On the plane:

- Don't stow your carry-on luggage under your seat if that will restrict your movement.
- Flex your calves and rotate your ankles every 20–30 minutes.
- Walk up and down the aisle every two hours or more frequently.
- Sleep only for short periods.
- Do not take sleeping pills.
- Drink lots of water to avoid dehydration.
- Avoid alcohol, caffeine, and diet soda.
- Wear elastic flight socks or support stockings.
- Don't let your stockings or clothing roll up or constrict your legs.
- Take deep breaths frequently throughout your flight.

The Straight Dope on Pharmaceuticals

- *True or false:* When traveling, it's okay to take small amounts of prescription drugs back into your home country.
- *True or false:* It's legal to order prescription drugs from reputable online pharmacies outside your home country.

Believe it or not—for many Western countries—the answer is false on both counts, though with some favorable caveats.

Many international travelers like to purchase their prescription medications less expensively while abroad. While that's *technically* illegal in the US and some other countries, consumer activists have turned the issue into a political hot potato. Consequently, at this writing, customs inspectors in the US are often reluctant to bust granny with her two vials of benazepril, and in most instances they turn a blind eye to folks entering the country with prescription medications purchased abroad. Thus, it's become a gray area, with customs inspectors empowered to use "general discretion" when prescription drugs are found. Most often, the offending pharmaceuticals are simply confiscated, and the traveler must decide whether it's worth all the red tape required to petition for their return.

The overwhelming majority of tourists carrying pharmaceuticals purchased abroad re-enter their home country with no trouble, usually unnoticed. The best advice is to use common sense. You're far less likely to be hassled for carrying a single prescription of amoxicillin than if your suitcase is bursting with enough tramadol to supply the streets of Los Angeles for a year. And as always, if you're carrying drugs that are illegal—prescription or otherwise—you may be subject to arrest, as well as seizure of your medications.

Similarly, it's *technically* illegal in the US and some other countries to purchase any pharmaceutical of any kind from any mail-order pharmacy outside the country. Again, highly vocal activists have prevailed politically in the US and elsewhere, and only a small fraction of prescription drugs purchased from foreign pharmacies is seized. In those cases, the pharmacies often double-ship the order, so the buyer usually doesn't even know the purchase was interrupted. (It's perfectly legal to purchase prescription drugs online from authorized mail-order pharmacies inside your home country.)

Again, until the laws change, you're advised to use good judgment. Purchase only from reputable pharmacies, using legitimate prescriptions from your physician—and anticipate the outside chance you'll be among the few every year inconvenienced by border seizures of prescription drugs.

For specifics about bringing controlled substances into the US, call 202 307.2414. US citizens can obtain additional information about traveling with medication from any FDA office or by writing to the US Food and Drug Administration, Division of Import Operations and Policy, Room 12-8 (HFC-170), 5600 Fishers Lane, Rockville, MD 20857. For further information on prescription drug rules and regulations, US citizens can contact the FDA's Center for Drugs at 888 INFO.FDA or visit www.fda.gov/cder. Citizens of other countries are encouraged to contact the appropriate government office for full rules and regulations.

Taking Drugs into Thailand

Can you carry drugs into Thailand? Yes, but limit drug transport to small bottles of medications prescribed by your doctor, carried in their original, labeled vials, and accompanied by their prescriptions. Carry with you a letter signed by your doctor that explains the reason why you need a particular medication. Antidrug laws are stringent in Thailand, and penalties for possession of illicit drugs are harsh. Don't risk being stopped in customs with an unlabeled bottle of a narcotic or psychotropic substance.

CHECKLIST 7: *What Does My Travel Companion Need to Do?*

A person who accompanies a health traveler gives a great gift. Here are some questions for potential companions to answer before they commit themselves to accompanying a health traveler abroad.

TRAVEL COMPANION'S CONSIDERATIONS	Yes	No	Not Sure	Notes to Myself
Am I sure I want to go? Am I sure I'm up to the task? (If you hesitate in answering either question, you may want to reconsider.)				
Am I willing and able to take responsibility for handling details, such as obtaining visas and passports?				
Do I feel comfortable acting as an advocate for the health traveler at times when he or she may need assistance?				
Have we agreed on the costs of the trip and on who is responsible for paying what?				
Do I feel sufficiently confident about handling experiences and challenges in a foreign country, such as getting through airports, arranging for taxis, or finding addresses?				
Do the health traveler and I communicate well enough to identify problems and solve them together amicably?				
Am I prepared to listen to and record doctor's instructions and provide reminders for the health traveler when needed?				
Can I help the health traveler stay in touch with family, friends, and healthcare providers back home?				
Have I allowed for "down time" and time for myself during the medical travel?				
Do I have the patience to help the health traveler through what might be a long and difficult recovery period, both abroad and back home?				

Thailand's Most Popular Medical Destinations

Having read Part One, you now have a fair idea of what it takes to be a smart and informed health traveler. At this point, chances are you've already reached a decision about your course of treatment, and you may be seriously considering Thailand as a destination for your medical care.

Part Two gives you an overview of Thailand's developments and achievements as an international medical hub and provides in-depth information about the leading healthcare establishments, as well as health travel agents, serving medical travelers to Thailand.

Introduction

In 2004 an earthquake in the Indian Ocean triggered a killer tsunami that devastated coastal areas throughout much of Southeast Asia. The disaster struck without warning, and only one nation in the region was prepared to provide the emergency medical care its citizens needed. That nation was Thailand. In response to this natural disaster, one of the deadliest in modern times, the Thais promptly delivered basic care in Phuket, Krabi, and Phang Nga and dispatched aid to their neighbors, Indonesia and Sri Lanka. Emergency food, water, and medical supplies were distributed so efficiently that foreign aid teams who rushed to Thailand found themselves with little left to do.

Thailand was able to respond rapidly and effectively for two reasons: a strong economy and a well-developed healthcare infrastructure. Both of those factors are as important to the health traveler as they are to local residents, and they are among the reasons why Thailand is often touted as the birthplace of medical tourism.

Strong Economy

Thailand's official status as a developing nation may come as a surprise to anyone who has ever fought rush-hour traffic in Bangkok or relaxed in a luxury hotel in Phuket. Although the nation's primary economic base lies in agriculture, industrialization is widespread, and Thailand boasts the highest gross domestic product (GDP) and the lowest poverty index (less than 10 percent) in the region. On the Human Development Index—a composite score of life expectancy at birth, adult literacy rate, mean years of schooling, and GDP per capita—Thailand scores highest in the region.

Economic growth has been strong and nearly constant in Thailand for more than 20 years. Between 1990 and 2006, Thailand's GDP more than tripled, despite a downturn in world economies in 1997–1998. Real growth in Thailand's GDP averages about 5 percent a year, driven largely by a strong export sector. Thailand's international trade nearly tripled between 1990 and 2003. The country enjoys a brisk export trade in pharmaceuticals (up by a factor of 10 since 1989), and a number of foreign drug companies operate manufacturing plants in Thailand.

Thailand, a middle-income country, contributes nearly as much to international assistance (as a proportion of its income) as do the world's richest countries. In the 2003 fiscal year, for example, its aid to other nations worked out at 0.13 percent of GDP (compared to 0.15 percent for the United States and 0.2 percent for Japan). Nearly all of Thailand's assistance goes to its less-developed neighbors, Myanmar (Burma), Lao PDR (Laos), and Cambodia. Assistance is provided directly in the construction of roads, bridges, and power stations, and indirectly through liberal polices that promote trade and open markets for exports.

Change runs rapid and deep in Thailand, and the Thais are quick to embrace technology—so quick that some experts predict Thailand will be ranked among the developed nations by 2030.

The Health of the Thai People

Since the 1980s, the health of the Thai people has vastly improved. Infant mortality has dropped from a high of 84.3 per thousand live births in 1964 to 16.3 in 2007. Vaccine-preventable deaths have dropped by as much as 90 percent, because Thailand achieves nearly a 99 percent immunization rate for children younger than one year.

Life expectancy at birth is now estimated at near-Western norms of 67.9 years for males and 75 years for females. As a result of reduced birth and death rates, the Thai population is aging. The percentage of people older than 60 is rising, and the aged are expected to constitute nearly 16 percent of the population by the year 2020.

As Thailand's economy has grown increasingly modern and Western, so has the lifestyle of its people—with all the health problems that ensue. Environmental pollution, stress, fast food, substance abuse, and sedentary occupations are bringing with them a growing burden of coronary artery disease, heart disease, diabetes, and lung disorders. Like its counterparts in developed nations, the Thai Ministry of Public Health is pursuing a five-pronged strategy for health promotion: exercise, diet, emotional development, disease reduction, and environmental health.

The ministry runs public awareness campaigns for the prevention and control of cardiovascular disease, particularly hypertension. Thailand is a nation of smokers, at least among the men—some 40 percent still smoke—but smoking dropped by about one-quarter between 1986 and 2001. Thailand has also taken major steps toward combating HIV/AIDS, which, in 2006, was the nation's leading cause of death. In 2003 the Ministry of Public Health implemented universal access to antiretroviral drugs for all HIV/AIDS patients.

Safe sex campaigns have been well received, as have family planning initiatives. Nearly 80 percent of Thailand's married women use contraceptives. As a result, Thailand's annual population growth rate dropped from 2.65 percent in 1980 to 0.8 percent in 2001. Such campaigns can be effective because the Thais are an educated people; the adult literacy rate is expected to reach 97 percent in the year 2010.

Thailand's Healthcare System

Thailand spends about 3.5 percent of its GDP on healthcare, a proportion that's comparatively low. However, its annual per capita expenditure of about US$260 per person compares favorably with other countries in the region. From 1992 to 1997, the share of total government expenditure devoted to health increased from 5.9 percent to 7.7 percent. The government's health budget has continued to rise steadily since 2001—the year that Thailand instituted a massive and rapid overhaul of its healthcare program with "the 30 Baht Scheme," which provides every citizen with primary healthcare for about 88 US cents per doctor visit.

The Thais had been debating a change in their healthcare system for many years, but when action was at last taken, it was taken immediately and universally, using a double-barreled approach. First, some 19 million people who had previously been without health insurance were immediately covered under a nationalized plan. Second, public funding shifted dramatically away from tertiary care in major urban hospitals and flowed to primary care in rural areas, where two-thirds of Thailand's population resides.

Today universal health insurance coverage reaches more than 75 percent of the population in all 75 provinces of Thailand. Public and private hospitals and clinics serve Thai citizens and international medical travelers in ever-growing numbers. Public facilities treated nearly 6 million inpatients in 2001, an increase of about 8 percent over the previous year—and private facilities treated 1.7 million inpatients, a single-year increase of a whopping 34 percent.

The Birth of Medical Travel

The Chinese say that within every crisis lies an opportunity, and that's exactly the situation Thailand faced in implementing a national healthcare plan. While providing care for many previously underserved sectors of the population, the reallocation in health funding caused problems for large, urban hospitals staffed largely with specialists. Tertiary-care hospitals faced a massive challenge in retraining staff and redirecting resources toward primary care. Despite the fact that 95 percent of Thailand's doctors work in cities and 79 percent work in tertiary care, large urban hospitals lost income and faced mounting deficits as government support shifted toward primary care in rural areas.

But from those problems sprang a benefit: *Thailand had surplus medical technology and specialist expertise to offer the world.*

Technology. Hospitals in large Thai cities are among the best equipped anywhere, due in large part to an investment boom through the 1980s and 1990s. During that period, medical technologies were freely imported into Thailand with duty exemptions, and the acquisition of medical equipment skyrocketed, especially in large urban centers. The imported value of medical equipment rose by 12.4 percent annually between 1991 and 2003. The result was an overabundance of medical equipment—at one time Bangkok had more computed tomography (CT) scanners per capita than the entire UK did. The investment in such big-ticket equipment has slowed since the economic downturn of 1997–1998. Nevertheless, Thailand is still way ahead of most of its Asian neighbors in medical technology.

Specialty care. Before the end of World War II, all physicians in Thailand were generalists, providing the sorts of services that Western countries label general or family practice. Starting in the 1950s, however, many Thai medical graduates sought post-graduate specialty training overseas, especially in the US. The Thai Medical Council, which is the national medical accrediting and licensing body, was established in the 1960s and began to approve specialty training and certification. After that, the number of medical school graduates who became general practitioners fell, while the number of specialists grew. In the 1970s and 1980s, large numbers of graduating Thai medical students relocated to the US and other countries to continue their education. At the same time, Thailand saw an increase in its number of private hospitals built to international standards. Many doctors moved from public to private facilities; today one in every five doctors in Thailand works at a private institution.

A new era. By the late 1990s, Thailand was ready to offer its medical services to the world. Thailand had a head start on serving international clients, because its doctors and hospitals had long been caring for an expatriate population numbering in the hundreds of thousands in metropolitan Bangkok. This multi-racial and highly demanding mix of resident foreigners provided a solid training ground for what was to come, and come it did. A buyers' market, Thai medicine offered high quality at low prices, and medical travelers flocked to Bangkok and Phuket for everything from hip replacements to facelifts, at costs 60–90 percent lower than back home.

Rising international tensions following the airplane bombing of New York's World Trade Center on September 11, 2001, drove many Middle Eastern medical travelers away from their traditional destinations in the US and the UK—and they traveled instead to Thailand. Today more than a million medical travelers visit Thailand every year. Officials at just one Thai hospital, Bumrungrad International, estimate that their hospital treats more than 1,500 international patients from more than 100 countries every day.

Thai Traditional Medicine

No discussion of Thai healthcare would be complete without a mention of Thai traditional medicine, an ancient blend of massage, herbal medicine, and spiritual healing that traces its roots back to the famous Buddhist temple at Wat Pho, believed to be the site of Thailand's first medical school and the birthplace of traditional Thai massage. Although traditional medicine fell into disrepute throughout much of the twentieth century, it made a strong comeback in the 1990s, and today many countries, including Thailand, are attempting to restore the best of traditional practices as a complement to modern scientific medicine.

Twenty-eight agencies in Thailand have formed the Federation of Thai Traditional Medicine, a network that aims to conserve and protect these age-old concepts and practices. The federation's museum, established in 2003, collects and analyzes the knowledge and methods of traditional medicine. Controlled experimentation evaluates the effectiveness of the herbs and extracts that have been used for millennia. It's a big job: about 4,000 herbs are eligible for investigation.

Several herbal preparations have already met the challenge of double-blind scientific testing, and the Ministry of Public Health now includes 28 items from Thai traditional medicine on its official list of general household medicines. Eleven types of herbal capsules, teas, creams, and lotions are manufactured by the Government Pharmaceutical Organization. Today about one-fifth of Thailand's health facilities—more than 2,300 hospitals and clinics—offer traditional medicine in some form. Examples include *plygesal* (a topical anti-inflammatory cream), *phaya yo* (a topical cream for shingles), *khamin chan* (curcumin capsules, an immune-boosting anti-inflammatory made from turmeric), and *fa thalai chon* (capsules prescribed for sore throat, fever, and diarrhea). Traditional medicine is made all the more effective by Thai hospitality, which some say is the finest in the world.

Thailand: A World-Class Medical Destination

Why is Thailand a prime destination for the medical traveler? Quality is high, prices are low, and access to care is often immediate, even without an appointment—not to mention the warmth of Thai hospitality, which can make even the most arduous medical procedure bearable, perhaps even pleasant.

Thailand is home to some 1,265 hospitals; of those, 309 are private hospitals, 83 of them in Bangkok. Private hospitals now represent 40 percent of all hospital beds in the Thai capital. Thailand has more than 19,000 physicians and 100,000 nurses in active practice. The nation's ten qualified medical colleges produce about 3,800 graduates yearly. Its 20 nursing schools graduate about 3,000 nurses annually, who have completed a minimum of four years' baccalaureate training (as compared to countries in which a nursing license may be obtained in two years). Each year a third of the graduating nurses earn masters or doctorate degrees.

Many Thai physicians undertake postgraduate education overseas and return to Thailand experienced in specialized services, such as cardiac surgery or cancer treatment. Bumrungrad International Hospital, for example, boasts more than 200 physicians who are board certified in the US, plus a large number who have trained in the UK, Germany, Australia, Belgium, Japan, and elsewhere.

In 2002 Thailand became home to Asia's first JCI-accredited hospital: Bumrungrad International in Bangkok, which has since had its accreditation renewed twice—in 2005 and 2008. Thailand now offers medical travelers six additional JCI-accredited facilities:

✦ Bangkok Hospital Medical Center, Bangkok (accredited 2007)

✦ Samitivej Srinakarin Hospital, Bangkok (accredited 2007)

✦ Samitivej Sukhumvit Hospital, Bangkok (accredited 2007)

✦ Samitivej Sriracha Hospital, Chonburi (accredited 2008)

✦ Bangkok Nursing Home Hospital, Bangkok (accredited 2009)

✦ Bangkok Hospital Phuket, Phuket (accredited 2009)

We profile these and 11 other health travel destinations in the next section, "Selected Hospitals and Clinics."

Selected Hospitals and Clinics

In this section we feature 18 hospitals; 16 are headquartered in Bangkok and two in Phuket.

Bangkok Adventist Hospital

430 Phitsanulok Road
Dusit
Bangkok, THAILAND 10300
Tel: 66 2 282.1100
Fax: 66 2 280.0441
Email: info.bangkok@mission-hospital.org
Web: www.mission-hospital.org

Bangkok Adventist Hospital, widely known among the Thais as the Mission Hospital, is owned and operated by the Christian Medical Foundation of the Seventh-day Adventists as part of the worldwide Adventist Healthcare Network. This hospital traces its history back to the modest Bangkok Mission Clinic, a 12-bed inpatient facility plus outpatient service established in 1937; it was officially renamed Bangkok Adventist Hospital in 1973. In 1983 a new wing was added onto the original building to expand outpatient, surgical, and examination facilities. In 1987 a new building was opened to provide beds for obstetric and pediatric patients, to house a new food and bakery service, and to accommodate additional parking.

Today Bangkok Adventist is a 185-bed hospital admitting more than 6,000 inpatients and treating nearly 200,000 outpatients annually; about 1,500 each year are international patients. The hospital currently has 450 employees and about 80 medical staff. Its imaging department utilizes x-ray, spiral computed tomography (CT), ultrasound, fluoroscopy, mammography, densitometry, and electrocardiography (EKG). One of the hospital's specialties is minimally invasive surgery, and its operating theater can accommodate five patients. The intensive care unit has beds for eight.

Other services include acupuncture, physical therapy, dialysis, hydrotherapy, testing for exercise stress and pulmonary function, and counseling for lifestyle management, including diabetes control and nutritional support. Bangkok Adventist's **International Travel Medicine Clinic** provides travel advice and vaccinations, treats tropical diseases, and tests blood for diagnosis of travel-related illnesses.

Bangkok Adventist maintains doctors on its wards 24/7. Admissions and ambulance services are always available, too, as are interpreters for English, Japanese, and Mandarin. Besides admitting and treating patients at the hospital, Bangkok Adventist runs an x-ray-equipped mobile clinic for charitable medical outreach.

Specialty Centers

✦ Allergy Clinic

✦ Breast Clinic

✦ Center for Health Promotion and Lifestyle Management

✦ Dental Center

✦ Gastrointestinal Clinic

✦ Hearing Center

✦ Hemodialysis Unit

✦ International Travel Medicine Clinic

✦ Skin and Laser Clinic

Bangkok Christian Hospital

124 Silom Road
Bangrak
Bangkok, THAILAND 10500
Tel: 66 2 235.1000; 66 2 233.6981
Fax: 66 2 236.2911
Email: info@bkkchristianhosp.th.com
Web: www.bkkchristianhosp.th.com

The Western missionaries who traveled to Thailand two centuries ago set out to spread the Christian faith and heal the sick. The local people called their visitors *mo*, which means "doctor."

Dr. Dan Beach Bradley from Marcellus, New York, was known as Mo Bradley to the people of Bangkok in 1835. He performed surgery, administered smallpox vaccine, and even translated a textbook of midwifery. The Presbyterian Mission Dr. Bradley established in 1840 was the beginning of Bangkok Christian Hospital, which was officially inaugurated by the Thai prime minister in 1949.

Since then Bangkok Christian has grown considerably. A three-story building opened in 1957 to serve the outpatient department, dentistry unit, laboratory, pharmacy, and chapel, and a new operating theater opened in 1961. In 1970 a staff dormitory was built, along with a modern kitchen and cafeteria; an office building and parking structure were added soon after. In 1981 an additional 13-story structure was named the Mo Bradley Building, in honor of the hospital's founder. A new inpatient building opened in 1987.

Bangkok Christian offers the full range of general medical services along with some specialties. The **Health Screening Center** provides package pricing for diagnostic and preventive tests ranging from lumbar spine exams to hernia assessment. A special health screening package available for people over the age of 45 includes basic blood tests (liver, kidney, blood counts, and lipid profile), EKG, chest x-ray, a prostate-specific antigen (PSA) test for males, and a Pap test for females.

The hospital's **Dental Care Center** is staffed with specialists in endodontics, oral surgery, pedodontics, and prosthodontics. Services include cosmetic dentistry, dentures, gum disease treatment, implants, oral and maxillofacial surgery, orthodontics, and root canal.

Bangkok Christian's **International Refractive Center** performs LASIK eye surgery. Other special services are offered in the hospital's **EEG and Sleep Laboratory** and the **Skin Care and Laser Center.**

Bangkok Hospital Medical Center

2 Soi Soonvijai 7
New Phetchaburi Road
Bangkapi, Huai Khwang
Bangkok, THAILAND 10310
Tel: 66 2 310.3000; 66 2 310.3344
Fax: 66 2 310.3327; 66 2 755.1310
Email: info@bangkokhospital.com
Web: www.bangkokhospital.com

The flagship of the mammoth Dusit Medical Group, which is Southeast Asia's largest private hospital network, Bangkok Hospital Medical Center (BMC) is one of the most technologically sophisticated healthcare centers in the world. The four main hospitals and numerous specialized clinics on the BMC campus are equipped with diagnostic and treatment facilities not generally available at local hospitals. Open since 1971, this 500-bed medical center received JCI accreditation in 2007, and it has an ongoing reputation for excellence. It is affiliated with the Barbara Ann Karmanos Cancer Institute in Detroit, Michigan, as well as the University of Baguio in the Philippines and Srinakharinwirot University in Bangkok.

BMC employs more than 650 full-time and consulting physicians, 700 nurses, and numerous teams of support technicians and specialists. Altogether, staff members speak a total of 28 languages. BMC operates in four main hospital buildings: Bangkok International Hospital, Bangkok Heart Hospital, Bangkok Hospital, and Wattanasoth Cancer Hospital, with two supporting buildings for dentistry and rehabilitation. The medical center's five major foci are cardiology, gastroenterology, neurology, oncology, and orthopedics. The three procedures most frequently performed at BMC are coronary bypass surgery, joint replacement, and percutaneous coronary intervention.

BMC's **Bangkok International Hospital** was the first Thai medical center to serve international patients. Its **International Medical Center** improved and expanded its services in 2002, and it now serves more than 150,000 patients annually from more than 60 countries—about 3,000 of these patients travel from the US and Canada. Sixteen specialized centers, ranging from orthopedics to neurology to cardiology, have brought together internationally trained physicians and state-of-the-art medical technology to attract visitors from all parts of the world.

The International Medical Center's team of 60 specialists helps overseas visitors overcome cultural and language barriers and also provides a host of other support services, including visa assistance, airport pickup, around-the-clock contact for medical assessments, advice on treatment options and doctors' appointments, arrangements for special diets, shopping and sightseeing tours, and liaison assistance with embassies, international organizations, and insurance claims.

BMC's **Bangkok Heart Hospital** is Thailand's first and only dedicated private heart hospital. Staffed by personnel who deal with nearly every heart condition, it is equipped with the most advanced technology for diagnostics, interventional cardiology, cardiac surgery, and rehabilitation. Frequently performed procedures include cardiac magnetic resonance imaging (MRI), CT, angiography, adult stem cell therapies, radiofrequency ablation (RFA), pacemaker implantation, and an all-artery cardiac bypass surgery. The hospital's da Vinci robotic surgery system is used in a variety of minimally invasive surgical procedures.

BMC's **Wattanasoth Cancer Hospital** is the only dedicated private oncology hospital in Thailand. It boasts state-of-the-art technologies that include positron emission tomography (PET) and CT scanning for fast and accurate diagnosis, NOVALIS for intensity-modulated radiotherapy (IMRT) and radiosurgery, and Gamma Knife for radiosurgery of the brain.

The 12 neurologists and 14 neurosurgeons on staff at BMC's **Bangkok Neuroscience Center** treat a host of diseases and traumas, including headache, dizziness, and vertigo; stroke and its aftermath; seizures; Parkinson's disease and related disorders; Alzheimer's disease; brain and spinal cord injury and tumors; neuromuscular diseases; paresthesia of the limbs, trunk, and face; developmental disorders; and genetic anomalies. Specialties within the center include clinics for stroke and cardiovascular disorders, pain, epilepsy, movement disorders, and neurogenetics. Its neurosurgeons also specialize in cerebral hemorrhage, aneurysms, head trauma, and skull-base and spinal surgery.

The Neuroscience Center's high-tech testing and instrumentation inventory includes CT, MRI, cerebral angiography, electroencephalography (EEG) monitoring, brainstem auditory evoked response, somatosensory evoked response, neurosonology carotid ultrasound, transcranial Doppler, and a spinal cord stimulation drug-infusion system. And by deploying the Gamma

Knife, the center's neurosurgeons can reach deep-seated brain lesions without the risks of open-skull surgery, as the hundreds of precisely targeted cobalt gamma radiation beams can painlessly "cut" through brain tumors, blood vessel malformations, and other abnormalities. Gamma Knife treatment enables the correction of disorders not currently treatable using more conventional procedures; furthermore, patients experience less discomfort and have greatly shortened recovery periods.

Various amenities from concierge services to luxury accommodations are available on the BMC campus, ensuring that every visitor's stay is comfortable. BMC's patient rooms rival those in the best US hospitals and include a guest sofa-bed for a companion, personal telephone for international calls, microwave oven, refrigerator, personal safe, free Internet access, free English-language newspaper, and an inpatient library.

Bangkok Hospital Specialty Centers

✦ Acupuncture and Acupressure Clinic

✦ Allergy and Asthma Center

✦ Antiaging Medicine Center

✦ Bangkok Neuroscience Center

✦ Breast Center

✦ Chest and Respiratory Care Center

✦ Child Health Center

✦ Comprehensive Spine Center

✦ Dental Center

+ Diabetes and Endocrine Center

+ Ear, Nose, and Throat Center

+ Endoscopy Center

+ Eye Center

+ Fertility Center

+ GI and Liver Center

+ Golfer Health Center

+ Hair Restoration Clinic

+ Health Promotion Center

+ Hyperbaric Oxygen Therapy Center

+ Internal Medicine Clinic

+ Kidney Center

+ LASIK Center

+ Neurosurgical Gamma Center

+ Obstetrics and Gynecology Clinic

+ Orthopedic Center

+ Rehabilitation Center

+ Skin and Aesthetics Center

+ Surgery Clinic

+ Trauma Center

+ Travel Medicine Clinic

+ Urological Center

Bangkok Heart Hospital Specialty Centers

✦ Cardiac Rehabilitation Clinic

✦ Heart Failure Clinic

✦ Preventive Cardiology Clinic

✦ Vascular Center

Achievements and Awards

✦ Asia's Top 200 Small and Midsize Companies, *Forbes*

✦ Hospital Accreditation, Ministry of Public Health

✦ Best Service Provider, Prime Minister's Export Award, 2001

✦ First Place, Integration of Quality Improvement Projects by Using the Standard Requirements of Hospital Accreditation and Brand Management, Hospital Management Asia Awards, 2002

✦ Asian Hospital Management Awards, 2002, 2006, and 2007

✦ Telemedicine for the Mobile Society (TEMOS) Partner Certification, 2007

✦ European Aero Medical Institute (EURAMI) Accreditation, 2008

✦ Business of the Year Award, Australian-Thai Chamber of Commerce, 2008

Bangkok International Dental Center

This dental center operates two locations:

Bangkok International Dental Center Main Headquarters

157 Ratchadaphisek Road
Din Daeng
Bangkok, THAILAND 10400
Tel: 66 2 692.4433
Fax: 66 2 248.6196
Email: contact@bangkokdentalcenter.com
Web: www.bangkokdentalcenter.com

BIDC@Siam Square

Sukhumvit Office
205/2-3 Phyathai Road
Pathumwan
Bangkok, THAILAND 10330
Tel: 66 2 658.4774
Fax: 66 2 658.4868
Email: contact@thailanddental.com
Web: www.bangkokdentalcenter.com

Formerly known as Bangkok Dental Group, the main Bangkok International Dental Center (BIDC) facility and its BIDC@Siam Square branch jointly provide more than 25 treatment rooms and the services of more than 70 dentists and dental specialists, many of whom have graduated from universities in the UK, the Americas, Australia, Singapore, and Hong Kong. BIDC's dentists continue their training through courses conducted at BIDC clinics and at other institutions.

The main BIDC headquarters in the Din Daeng district is a more than 48,000-square-foot (4,500-square-meter) complex consisting of a seven-story dental clinic, a 30-room hotel, a bank, a restaurant, and a coffee shop. The clinic has its own onsite laboratory specializing in dental implants. BIDC was the first center in Thailand to offer the SLActive Straumann Dental Implant System, as well as the Bone Level Straumann Dental Implant System, which was only recently launched worldwide.

BIDC provides many amenities for its patients, including free high-speed Internet terminals and cable television, as well as private conference and consultation rooms. Contact the clinic before you travel for recommendations on accommodations, because BIDC also offers special corporate rates for guests at selected hotels near its clinics. Best of all, dental patients accustomed to US and European prices for reconstructive work such as implants are in for a pleasant surprise: you might pay US$1,500 for a porcelain crown at home—but at BIDC, you'll pay something like US$220–470 (7,500–16,000 baht). Maybe that's why BIDC treats more than 6,000 international patients each year, 2,200 of them from Canada and the US.

Specialties

✦ Aesthetic dentistry

✦ Dental implants

✦ Endodontics

✦ General dentistry

✦ Oral surgery

✦ Orthodontics

✦ Pedodontics

✦ Periodontics

✦ Preventive dentistry

✦ Prosthodontics

Bangkok Nursing Home Hospital

9/1 Convent Road
Silom, Bangrak
Bangkok, THAILAND 10500
Tel: 66 2 686.2700
Fax: 66 2 632.0579
Email: info@bnhhospital.com; itmc@bnh.co.th
(for international travelers)
Web: www.bnhhospital.com

Don't be fooled by the name—Bangkok Nursing Home Hospital (BNH) is not a nursing home in the American sense of the word. Founded in the nineteenth century as a hospital for expatriates living in Thailand, today BNH is a modern, full-service, 120-bed hospital that received its JCI accreditation in 2009. More than 23,000 international patients visit BNH annually, some 4,000 of them from the US and Canada. As one of the smaller members of the Dusit Medical Group, BNH prides itself on intimacy and personal attention for its patients.

With a high in vitro fertilization (IVF) success rate, the hospital's **Bangkok IVF Center** is popular among medical travelers. BNH also operates a special center for spinal and orthopedic surgery. Since opening in 2005, the **Spine Center** has performed more than 200 complex surgeries, nearly half of them for international patients. BNH was the first hospital in Thailand to offer total artificial disc replacement (TADR) and DIAM implantation (a new technology for posterior stabilization of the spine). The surgical team has also implanted over 100 disc prostheses, a rate higher than some centers in the US or EU.

Specialty Centers

+ Bangkok IFV Center
+ Cardiac Care Unit
+ Checkup Center
+ Critical Care Unit
+ Dental Clinic
+ Diabetes and Hormone Clinic
+ Ear, Nose, and Throat Clinic
+ Emergency and Trauma Center
+ Endocrinology and Nephrology Clinic
+ Gastrointestinal and Liver Clinic
+ Geriatric Care Center
+ Heart Center
+ Hemodialysis Unit
+ International Travel Medicine Clinic
+ Ladies' Urinary Care Center
+ Men's Health Center

✦ Nutrition Clinic

✦ Ophthalmology Department

✦ Pain Clinic

✦ Pediatrics Department

✦ Radiology Department

✦ Rehabilitation and Physical Therapy Department

✦ Shoulder and Joint Center

✦ Spine Center

✦ Women's Health Center

Achievements and Awards

✦ PR and Brand Management, Asian Hospital Management Award, Faber Medi-Serve Group, 2004

✦ Most Recognized Service, Prime Minister's Export Award, 2004

✦ Best Services, AustCham Thailand Business Award, Australian Chamber of Commerce, 2007

✦ Best Professional Services, Export Services Company, Business Excellence Award, Thai-Canadian Chamber of Commerce, 2007

✦ Hospital Accreditation, Ministry of Public Health, 2008

Bumrungrad International Hospital

33 Sukhumvit 3 (Soi Nana Nua)
Wattana
Bangkok, THAILAND 10110
Tel: 66 2 667.1000
Fax: 66 2 667.2525
Email: info@bumrungrad.com
Web: www.bumrungrad.com

Established in 1980, Bumrungrad International Hospital is the largest private hospital in Southeast Asia. It serves more than a million patients per year, including more than 400,000 international patients who visit from 190 countries; more than 30,000 of those medical travelers come from the US or Canada. In 2002 Bumrungrad became Asia's first hospital to obtain JCI accreditation, and it has been reaccredited twice since then. At this writing, it is one of Thailand's seven JCI-accredited hospitals. It was also the first Asian hospital to receive JCI disease-specific accreditations for its stroke and heart attack programs.

Bumrungrad recently opened its **International Clinic** building, and most of the hospital's outpatient clinics moved there in 2009. Doctor's rooms have instant computer access to patient records, lab results, and medical images. In the **International Medical Coordination Office,** staff members provide coordination, support, and help for patients coming from outside Thailand for medical treatment. A food court, Starbucks café, and bookshop welcome visitors, and the Napa Lounge offers a relaxing break for members of the hospital's new Healthy Living Club. Each outpatient floor features an education center with informative displays and take-home materials. Each clinic floor provides cashier and pharmacy counters for convenient, one-stop service.

Bumrungrad's 554-bed inpatient facility provides a full range of tertiary healthcare services. Its 19 operating rooms are equipped for most general surgery procedures and surgical specialties. Some of these procedures are minimally invasive, including cardiothoracic, laser, ophthalmologic, orthopedic, otorhinolaryngologic (ear, nose, and throat), transplantation, and urologic surgeries.

The hospital's 34 clinical specialties include endocrinology (diabetes and metabolism), nephrology (kidneys), neurology, and nutrition. Bumrungrad's **Heart Center** offers pacemaker implantation, invasive and noninvasive procedures for congenital heart disease, valvoplasty (balloon valve treatment), valve replacement, and coronary artery bypass graft (CABG). The hospital's **Horizon Regional Cancer Center** employs such advanced techniques as image-guided radiotherapy (IGRT) and high-dose brachytherapy. Orthopedic procedures, such as hip replacement and resurfacing, are also popular among Bumrungrad's international patients.

Of Bumrungrad's nearly 1,100 physicians, surgeons, and consultants, approximately 200 are US board certified. Staff members speak Thai and English. Interpreters are available for Arabic, Bengali, Chinese, French, German, Japanese, Khmer, Korean, and Vietnamese. Directed by a US-trained medical director, Bumrungrad International sponsors an active continuing medical education program for its physicians, who also participate in clinical research through the **Bumrungrad International Clinical Research Center.**

The hospital commissions an independent research firm to conduct a customer satisfaction survey each year. In the most recent survey, nine out of ten international patients reported being satisfied with their experience and said they would recommend the hospital—and one of the reasons is transparent pricing. Bumrungrad's Web site features a REALCOST service, which shows the low, high, and median bills that patients paid for 45 different procedures in the previous calendar year; it also displays package prices for straightforward, routine, and uncomplicated procedures. To see how it works, check out www .bumrungrad.com/realcost.

Bumrungrad offers two residential facilities for recovering patients and their family members. The first, Bumrungrad Hospitality Suites, is a 51-room serviced apartment complex located within walking distance of the hospital. The property has a range of options from studio apartments to three-bedroom suites, for daily, weekly, and monthly rental. All rooms come with complete support services, including maid and concierge service, 24-hour security, and an appointment desk linked directly to the hospital.

The second, Bumrungrad Residences, is a 74-room serviced apartment complex connected to the main hospital building by an air-conditioned, elevated walkway. It's within easy walking distance of restaurants, shopping, and entertainment venues, as well as Bangkok's elevated-train service. Shared facilities include a swimming pool, Jacuzzi, sauna, and steam room. (No medical personnel are on duty in either facility.)

Specialty Centers

✦ Allergy Center

✦ Breast Care Center

✦ Children's Center

✦ Dental Center

✦ Diabetes Center

✦ Diagnostic and Therapeutic Center

✦ Dialysis Center

✦ Digestive Disease Center

✦ Ear, Nose, and Throat Center

✦ Emergency Center

✦ Eye Center

✦ Eye Laser Refraction Center

✦ Fertility Center

✦ Health Screening Center

✦ Heart Center

✦ Horizon Regional Cancer Center

✦ Hyperbaric Oxygen Therapy Center

✦ Medical Clinics Center

✦ Men's Center

✦ Neurology Center

✦ Orthopedic Center

✦ Plastic Surgery Center

✦ Rehabilitation Center

✦ Skin Center

✦ Skin Laser Center

✦ Sleep Disorders Center

✦ Surgical Clinics Center

✦ Women's Center

Services Provided for International Patients

✦ The International Medical Coordination Office, staffed by seven doctors and 12 nurses, coordinates scheduling, treatment, and followup care.

✦ Customer service representatives speak English and Thai as well as Arabic, Bengali, Chinese, French, German, Japanese, Khmer, Korean, and Vietnamese. Interpretation in other languages can be arranged.

✦ One of Asia's top travel agencies, Diethelm Travel, has an office at Bumrungrad to arrange travel or local accommodations for patients and their families.

✦ Bumrungrad operates its own desk in the arrival area of Suvarnabhumi International Airport. Hospital staff members meet patients for plane-to-hospital VIP service.

✦ The Thai Immigration Bureau/Ministry of Interior processes visa extensions at the hospital weekly.

✦ Bumrungrad maintains offices in 21 countries: Angola, Australia, Bangladesh, Cambodia, Ethiopia, Germany, Hong Kong,

Kuwait, Mongolia, Myanmar, Nepal, New Zealand, Nigeria, Oman, Portugal, Seychelles, Sudan, Taiwan, Ukraine, Vietnam, and Yemen. Representatives in those offices work hard to ensure that patients receive the information and support they need.

Achievements and Awards

✦ Featured on CBS's *60 Minutes* and NBC's *Today Show* as a leader in medical travel

✦ Prime Minister's Export Award, 2002

✦ Best Small Cap Company Award, *Asiamoney,* 2004 and 2008

✦ First Place in quality and Fourth Place overall, Most-Admired Thai Companies, *Wall Street Journal Asia* readers, 2008

✦ Award of Excellence, Health Tourism–Oriented Medical Establishment, Thailand Tourism Awards, 2008

✦ Thailand's Most Innovative Company, Chulalongkorn University's School of Business, 2008

✦ Best Website for International Medical Travel, *Consumer Health* World Awards, Washington, DC, 2008

✦ Thailand Quality Class Recognition Award, 2008

Phyathai Group

This group shares the same email address and Web site:

Email: onestop@phyathai.com
Web: www.phyathai.com

Phyathai 1 Hospital

364/1 Sri-Ayutthaya Road
Ratchathewi
Bangkok, THAILAND 10400
Tel: 66 2 640.1111
Fax: 66 2 645.5488

Phyathai 2 Hospital

943 Phaholyothin Road
Samsennai, Phyathai
Bangkok, THAILAND 10400
Tel: 66 2 617.2444
Fax: 66 2 617.2499

Phyathai 3 Hospital

207/26 Phetchakasem Road
Pak Khlong, Phasri Charoen
Bangkok, THAILAND 10160
Tel: 66 2 467.1111
Fax: 66 2 467.6515

Phyathai Sriracha Hospital

90 Srirachanakhon 3 Road
Sriracha
Chonburi, THAILAND 20110
Tel: 66 38 77.0200
Fax: 66 38 77.0213

Phyathai 1 Hospital has established a reputation for minimally invasive neurosurgery, including brain surgery. The **Heart Center** at **Phyathai 2 Hospital** offers 24-hour surgical and nonsurgical treatment and medical care for patients with heart diseases. Phyathai 2 is also home to the **Musculoskeletal Center,** which provides medical care and surgery for bone, muscle, tendon, nerve, vessel, and joint disorders. **Phyathai 3** specializes in maternal and child health and offers assisted reproductive technologies and counseling. **Phyathai Sriracha Hospital** is about 60 miles (about 100 kilometers) from Bangkok, in the province of Chonburi. It offers all the specialties you might expect — and one you might not: travelers who are ill can call Phyathai Sriracha, and a doctor or nurse from the hospital will visit their hotel room.

Specialty Centers

+ Allergy Clinic
+ Checkup Center
+ Child Center
+ Cosmetic Center
+ Dental Center
+ Dermatology Clinic
+ Ear, Nose, and Throat Clinic
+ Eye Center
+ Gastrointestinal and Endoscopy Center

✦ Heart Center

✦ Internal Medicine Department

✦ LASIK Center

✦ Musculoskeletal Center

✦ Neurological Center

✦ Oncology Center

✦ Woman Center

Services Provided for International Patients

✦ Free consultation and medical advice via Internet

✦ Timely appointment scheduling

✦ Transportation arrangements, including airport pickup and ground or air ambulance

✦ Hotel or long-term lodging arrangements for patients and their families

✦ Advance financial and billing arrangements, including detailed estimates

✦ Preregistration and coordination of admission

✦ Personal escort to appointments and procedures

✦ Appointments for family members requesting routine or preventive medical care

✦ Special diets, including Western, Japanese, and Muslim food

✦ Business center for overseas calls and faxing

✦ Assistance with insurance

✦ Liaison service with embassies, international institutions, and other organizations

✦ Wireless Internet access and international television channels

Piyavate International Hospital

998 Rimkhlong Samsen Road
Bangkapi, Huai Khwang
Bangkok, THAILAND 10310
Tel: 66 2 625.6500
Fax: 66 2 625.6650
Email: imcc@piyavate.net
Web: www.piyavate.com

Piyavate (pronounced bee-yah-WAIT) International Hospital, a publicly owned healthcare services facility, began serving patients in 1993. This 26-story hospital houses nearly 300 inpatient beds and offers numerous medical specialties. Piyavate's **Advanced Dental Institute** provides services ranging from dental implants and cosmetic dentistry to oral surgery and braces. The hospital's **Aesthetic Surgery Institute** offers cosmetic plastic surgery and, through its **Romrawin Clinic,** comprehensive treatment for skin conditions, as well as antiaging skin care. In Piyavate's **Rehabilitation Center,** advanced equipment is utilized to provide patients with physical therapy and occupational rehabilitation. Treatments in the traditional **Chinese Medicine Center** include acupuncture, Chinese herbal medicine, and Tui Na massage. Piyavate also offers competitively priced physical exams and checkups, including a blood test, diabetes test, DNA test, and stress test, plus a breast and gynecological examination for women.

Specialties

✦ Alternative medicine

✦ Cardiology

✦ Dentistry

✦ Dermatology

✦ Ear, nose, and throat

✦ Emergency medicine

✦ Endocrinology

✦ Gastroenterology

✦ General medicine

✦ Gerontology

✦ Hematology

✦ Infectious disease

✦ Nephrology

✦ Neurology

✦ Oncology

✦ Ophthalmology

✦ Orthopedics

✦ Pediatrics

✦ Physical therapy and rehabilitation

✦ Plastic surgery

✦ Psychiatry

✦ Pulmonary medicine

✦ Radiology

✦ Rheumatology

✦ Surgery

✦ Urology

✦ Women's health

Specialty Centers

✦ Advanced Dental Institute

✦ Aesthetic Surgery Institute

✦ Bone and Joint Institute

✦ Chinese Medicine Center

✦ Neuroscience Center

✦ Oncology and Gene Therapy Center

✦ Perfect Heart Institute

✦ Perfect Woman Institute

✦ Rehabilitation Center

Services Provided for International Patients

✦ Medical consultation and advice

✦ Timely appointment scheduling

✦ Advance financial and billing arrangements, including detailed estimates

✦ Visa and flight preparation services

✦ Travel arrangements

✦ Transportation arrangements, including airport pickup and ground or air ambulance

✦ Personal escort to appointments and procedures

✦ Language interpretation: Arabic, Bengali, Burmese, Chinese, English, Filipino, Hindi, Italian, Japanese, Urdu, and Vietnamese

✦ Daily visits to inpatients by the international nurse coordinator and the international coordinator

✦ Preparation and transmission of medical documents

✦ Worldwide Assistance Insurance

Praram 9 Hospital

99 Soi Praram 9
Huai Khwang
Bangkok, THAILAND 10320
Tel: 66 2 202.9900
Fax: 66 2 248.8018
Email: info@praram9.com
Web: www.praram9.com

Praram 9 Hospital has been in operation since 1992. Employing more than 200 physicians, it offers a comprehensive range of medical services through its various departments and specialized centers.

Diagnostic and treatment services at the **Cardiovascular Institute** and **Cardiac Rehabilitation Center** include percutaneous transluminal coronary angioplasty (PTCA) and stent, cardiac catheterization, valvuloplasty, automatic implantable cardioverter defibrillator (AICD), radiofrequency catheter ablation, and more. The **Dental Clinic** provides everything from laser gum surgery to tooth whitening. The hospital's **Infertility Center** has achieved a high rate of successful pregnancies, while the **Kidney Transplant Institute** has achieved a success rate as high as those achieved in the US, Canada, and Western Europe.

Praram 9's **Orthopedic Center** specializes in the treatment of joint diseases and in bone and joint surgery. Modern diagnostic service using 4D-ultrasound technology and amniocentesis for detection of Down's syndrome is provided at the **Prenatal Diagnosis Center.** Physicians at this center also perform male and female sterilizations. The hospital's **Renal Center** frequently receives patients from overseas who need hemodialysis while traveling or visiting in Thailand.

Specialty Centers

✦ Allergy and Asthma Center

✦ Blastocyst Center

✦ Cardiac Rehabilitation Center

✦ Cardiovascular Institute

✦ Checkup Center

✦ Dental Center

✦ Digestive Disease Center

✦ Emergency Center

✦ Eye, Ear, Nose, and Throat Center

✦ Imaging Center

✦ Infertility Center

✦ Kidney Transplant Institute

✦ Medicine Center

✦ Obstetrics and Gynecology Center

✦ Orthopedic Center

✦ Pediatrics Center

✦ Prenatal Diagnosis Center

✦ Psychiatric Center

✦ Rehabilitation Center

✦ Renal Center

✦ Skin and Cosmetic Center

Services Provided for International Patients

✦ Arrangements for airline tickets

✦ Arrangements for airport pickup and dropoff

✦ Short-term and long-term lodging arrangements for patients and their families

✦ 24-hour language interpretation

✦ International menu

✦ Shuttle bus to Mass Rapid Transit (MRT) Phetchaburi Station

✦ Arrangements for tours and shopping trips

Achievements and Awards

✦ Research of the Year Award, Sixth Congress of the Asian Society of Transplantation (Singapore), 1999

✦ More kidney transplants performed at the Kidney Transplant Institute than any other private hospital in Thailand

Preecha Aesthetic Institute

Bangkok Mediplex, 2nd Floor, Unit 201–203
2/70 Sukhumvit 42
Phra Khanong, Khlong Toei
Bangkok, THAILAND 10250
Tel: 66 2 712.1111
Fax: 66 2 713.6500
Email: consult@pai.co.th
Web: www.pai.co.th

Preecha Aesthetic Institute (PAI) is headed by Dr. Preecha Tiewtranon, a leader in modern plastic, reconstructive, and aesthetic surgery. Former chairman of the plastic surgery unit of King Chulalongkorn University Medical School, he has served as president of the Plastic and Reconstructive Surgeons of Thailand and also as president of the Society of Aesthetic Surgeons of Thailand. As of 2005, Dr. Preecha had personally performed more than 30,000 cosmetic and plastic surgeries. As Bangkok's undisputed authority in gender reassignment, he has trained most of Thailand's qualified gender reassignment surgeons, and his techniques have become standard practice throughout the world. From 1980 to 2005, Dr. Preecha personally performed more than 3,500 gender reassignment and facial feminization surgeries.

PAI's modern hospital facility, located in the heart of Bangkok, offers a full range of dermatological treatments and plastic surgeries in its **Aesthetic Plastic Surgery Center** and **Dermatology and Laser Center.** The institute's staff of 30 includes practitioners who hold diplomas from the American Board of Surgery as well as surgeons who are board certified in the US,

Australia, and Thailand. PAI's services include cheekbone, facial, and jaw contouring; eye therapies, rhinoplasty, and various surgeries of the ear, lips, and chin; hair transplant and laser hair removal; and mammoplasty, labiaplasty, and vaginoplasty. Certain physicians at PAI specialize in body contouring, facial feminization, and gender reassignment surgery.

Specialties

+ Aesthetic plastic surgery: body contouring, skin rejuvenation, jaw surgery, mandibular angle resection, dimples, laugh line, gonioplasty, labiaplasty, pectoral implant, bone cement, calf implant

+ Gender reassignment surgery: male to female, breast, facial feminization surgery, Adam's apple/tracheal shaving, body contouring, female to male, gluteal implant

+ Penile enlargement: widening, lengthening by phalloplasty

Services Provided for International Patients

+ Travel and tour arrangements
+ Private consulting room
+ VIP lounge and waiting area
+ Pre-checkup room and post-op care room
+ Language interpretation
+ Post-operative care
+ Free portfolio

✢ Personal cell phone to use during recuperation in Thailand

✢ Private limousine (optional)

Ramkhamhaeng Hospital

2138 Ramkhamhaeng Road
Hua Mak, Bangkapi
Bangkok, THAILAND 10240
Tel: 66 2 374.0200
Fax: 66 2 374.0804
Email: info@ramhospital.com
Web: www.ramhospital.com

Ramkhamhaeng (pronounced ram-cam-HANG) Hospital sits at the center of one of Thailand's largest and most respected hospital groups. With 350 beds and seven sister hospitals, Ramkhamhaeng boasts the latest in imaging equipment, including MRI, ultrasound, and 64-slice CT. Modern diagnostic technology employed at the hospital's **Heart Center** includes echocardiography and Holter monitoring. Cardiac catheterization, CABG, PTCA, and stent implantation are frequently performed.

Specialties

✢ Heart diagnosis, treatment, surgery, and rehabilitation

✢ Hip and knee replacement

✢ IVF and embryo transfer (at neighboring Synphaet Hospital)

✢ Plastic surgery

Specialty Centers

✦ Checkup Clinic

✦ Dental Clinic

✦ Gender Reassignment Clinic

✦ Heart Center

✦ Hip Replacement Clinic

✦ Knee Replacement Clinic

✦ Laser Eye Surgery Clinic

✦ Oncology Clinic

✦ Sleep Clinic

Services Provided for International Patients

✦ Airport pickup and transfers

✦ English-speaking support staff

✦ Personal escort to appointments and procedures

Rutnin Eye Hospital

80/1 Sukhumvit 21 Road
Soi Asoke, Wattana
Bangkok, THAILAND 10110
Tel: 66 2 639.3399
Fax: 66 2 639.3311
Email: contact@rutnin.com
Web: www.rutnin.com

Rutnin Eye Hospital, founded in 1964 by Dr. Uthai Rutnin, was Thailand's first private hospital specializing exclusively in ophthalmology. Dr. Rutnin studied at Harvard University in Cambridge, Massachusetts, and was Thailand's first retinal specialist. He also founded and headed the Department of Ophthalmology at Ramathibodi Hospital, one of Thailand's largest teaching hospitals.

Today the hospital that bears his name employs 29 board-certified physicians and surgeons in every ophthalmologic subspecialty, including cornea, glaucoma, neuro-ophthalmology, oculoplastics, pediatric ophthalmology, vitreoretina, and excimer laser refractive surgery. Cross-referrals within the hospital ensure that every patient is seen by the appropriate subspecialist. English-speaking staff members welcome international patients. Rutnin's inpatient clinic is open seven days a week, and inpatients recover after surgery in the hospital's wards.

Specialty Centers

✦ Cataract Clinic

✦ Children's Eye Center and Orthoptic Clinic

✦ Cornea Transplanting and Anterior Segment Clinic

✦ Day Surgery Unit

✦ Glaucoma Clinic

✦ Lacrimal Clinic

✦ Laser Unit

✦ Low Vision Clinic

✦ Neuro-ophthalmology Clinic

✦ Ocular Prosthetics Clinic

✦ Oculoplastics Clinic

✦ Rutnin-Gimbel Excimer Laser Eye Center

✦ Uveitis Clinic

✦ Vitreoretina Clinic

Saint Louis Hospital

27 South Sathon Road
Bangkok, THAILAND 10120
Tel: 66 2 210.9999
Email: contact@saintlouis.or.th
Web: www.saintlouis.or.th

Saint Louis Hospital is a nonprofit general hospital occupying approximately 344,450 square feet (32,000 square meters) on South Sathon Road. After it was established in 1898 by Archbishop Louis Vey, Apostolic Vicar of the Roman Catholic Mission, the sisters of Saint Paul de Chartres were assigned to manage the hospital under the philosophy of "Where there is mercy, there is God."

Frequently performed procedures include digital heart catheterization, exercise stress testing, mammography, and bone densitometry. The hospital's operating room was imported ready-made from Germany, and experienced surgeons and anesthesiologists are on duty 24/7. The intensive care and cardiac care units maintain a central monitoring system. Patients' rooms are air-conditioned.

Saint Louis has been treating heart patients since 1979, and it was the first private hospital in Thailand to perform heart surgery successfully. Its **Heart Institute,** established in 1987, diagnoses and treats heart conditions and vascular diseases. Among the hospital's various other specialty centers is the **Dermatology and Skin Laser Center,** boasting the most comprehensive array of dermatological laser applications in Southeast Asia. Laser treatments correct congenital and other abnormalities and revitalize normal skin. The center's carbon dioxide laser is used for moles, warts, age spots, hard corns, skin cancers, and skin tumors; a pulse dye laser is used for red birthmarks, abnormal blood vessels, and scars; and a ruby laser is used for black birthmarks, Nevus of Ota birthmarks, and tattoo removal.

Saint Louis also operates a Thai Traditional Massage Center at the Saint Louis Medical Spa, located on the twenty-third floor of the Roipi Barameebun Building.

Specialty Centers

✦ Accident and Emergency Center

✦ Chinese Traditional Medicine Clinic

✦ Dental Center

✦ Department of Medicine

✦ Department of Obstetrics and Gynecology

✦ Department of Pediatrics

✦ Dermatology and Skin Laser Center

✦ Ear, Nose, and Throat Clinic

✦ Eye Clinic

✦ Gastrointestinal Clinic

✦ Gynecologic Oncology Clinic

✦ Health Checkup Center

✦ Heart Institute

✦ High Risk Pregnancy Clinic

✦ Infertility Clinic

✦ Menopausal Clinic (Golden Age Clinic)

✦ Nephrology Clinic and Hemodialysis Center

✦ Orthopedic Center

✦ Physical Rehabilitation Center

✦ Radiology Department

✦ Surgery Department

✦ Urology Center

✦ Women's Health Clinic

Samitivej Group

The Samitivej Group operates four hospitals in or near Bangkok. Three of them—Sukhumvit, Sriracha, and Srinakarin—are JCI accredited (denoted below with an asterisk).

*Samitivej Sukhumvit Hospital

133 Sukhumvit 49
Khlongtan Nua, Wattana
Bangkok, THAILAND 10110
Tel: 66 2 711.8000
Fax: 66 2 391.1290
Email: info@samitivej.co.th
Web: www.samitivejhospitals.com

In operation since 1979, Samitivej Sukhumvit Hospital currently has 270 beds, 87 examination suites, 400 full- and part-time physicians, 1,200 caregivers, and a full-service **International Patient Center.** Interpreters assist patients in Arabic, English, French, German, Japanese, and Korean, and the hospital's immigration counter assists foreigners with visa and other immigration requirements.

Sukhumvit is one of the few Thai hospitals to have received the Prime Minister's Award for Most Recognized Service (2004), and is accredited by Thailand's Institute of Hospital Quality Improvement and Accreditation. It has been designated by the

World Health Organization (WHO) as a "Baby-Friendly Hospital." American visitors will feel at home with a 7-Eleven, Starbucks, and ATMs on the ground level of the hospital. Sukhumvit treats 92,300 international patients annually, more than 16,000 of them from the US and Canada.

Sukhumvit's specialty centers include

+ **Eye Clinic:** specializes in general ophthalmology, pediatric ophthalmology and strabismus, retinal and vitreous conditions, glaucoma, oculoplastic reconstruction, and ocular oncology.

+ **Hemodialysis Department:** treats patients with acute or chronic renal failure. Certified by the Royal College of Physicians of Thailand, the department is known throughout the country for its success rate in kidney transplantation. Kidneys are received from the Thai Red Cross Organ Donation Center. Artificial kidney machines are also deployed for hemodialysis.

+ **Liver and Digestive Institute:** treats liver and other digestive abnormalities, including cirrhosis, fatty liver disease, pancreatitis, and infection of the bile duct and gallbladder. Specialty surgeries include liver transplantation as well as procedures on the liver, bile duct, gallbladder, esophagus, stomach, small intestine, and large intestine.

+ **Minimally Invasive Bone and Joint Center:** provides evaluation, diagnosis, and treatment for all bone- and joint-related ailments. The center's orthopedic surgeons treat broken bones, displaced joints, joint inflammation, slipped discs, and congenital malformations. They frequently perform microsurgery for the knee and shoulder as well as hip and knee replacements.

✦ **Plastic Surgery Clinic:** offers all types of cosmetic and reconstructive surgery, including rhinoplasty (nose), upper and lower blephaloplasty (eyelids), abdominal lipectomy (tummy tuck), facelift, liposuction, breast augmentation, chin augmentation, scar revision/repair, correction of congenital abnormalities, and post-mastectomy breast repair and reconstruction. UltraPulse and Sharplan carbon dioxide lasers are used to remove skin tags, warts, moles, and scars safely and effectively. Many procedures can be handled on an outpatient basis.

*Samitivej Sriracha Hospital

8 Soi Laemket
Cherm Chompon Road
Sriracha
Chonburi, THAILAND 20110
Tel: 66 38 32.0300
Fax: 66 38 31.2963
Email: marketing@ssh.samitivej.co.th
Web: www.samitivejhospitals.com

Samitivej Sriracha Hospital is located about 60 miles (100 kilometers) southeast of Bangkok. Since its opening more than a dozen years ago, this 150-bed hospital has become a key healthcare provider for corporations and industries on Thailand's Eastern seaboard. Sriracha's proximity to the resort towns of Pattaya and Rayong also attracts many tourists looking for quality healthcare facilities. The hospital has 15 intensive care units and six operating rooms. Its special services include the **Children's Clinic, Dental Clinic,** and **Wellness Center.** It acquired an MRI scanner in 2006.

*Samitivej Srinakarin Hospital

488 Srinakarin Road
Suan Luang
Bangkok, THAILAND 10250
Tel: 66 2 378.9000
Fax: 66 2 731.7044
Email: info.snch@samitivej.co.th
Web: www.samitivejhospitals.com

Samitivej Srinakarin Hospital is the group's newest addition, located on Bangkok's east side, a few minutes from the newly opened Suvarnabhumi International Airport. The 400-bed, 17-story main hospital building is surrounded by 21 acres (about 8.5 hectares) of landscaped gardens and fountains that foster an environment of tranquility not commonly found on the grounds of US hospitals.

Srinakarin's **Cancer Center** and **Oncology Clinic** focus on prevention, screening, diagnosis, and outpatient treatment. A full team of multilingual medical and radiation oncologists, physicists, technicians, and oncology and intravenous nurses render Bangkok's best in cancer treatment. The complete range of dental services and oral surgeries is offered at the hospital's **Dental Center,** including orthodontics, root canal, full and partial dentures, crowns and bridges, implants, extraction, bone graft surgery, and treatment of gum disease. Seven dental units, three x-ray operating suites, a panoramic x-ray machine, a laser system, and an intraoral camera make this center a state-of-the-art, one-stop shop, with no need for multiple trips to offsite labs.

Samitivej Srinakarin Children's Hospital

488 Srinakarin Road
Suan Luang
Bangkok, THAILAND 10250
Tel: 66 2 378.9000
Fax: 66 2 731.7044
Email: info.snch@samitivej.co.th
Web: www.samitivejhospitals.com

In 2003 the Samitivej Group opened Thailand's first—and today still the only—private hospital dedicated solely to children. Samitivej Srinakarin Children's Hospital offers highly specialized services, such as adolescent psychiatry at its **Bangkok Child Development Center,** Down's syndrome treatment at its **Bangkok Genetic Disorder Clinic,** weight control at the **Bangkok Weight Control Center,** and treatment for pediatric snoring at the **Bangkok Sleep Disorder Clinic.**

The hospital is well known for its **Bone Marrow Transplant Unit** and **Neonatal Intensive Care Unit.** In 2006 Samitivej Children's opened the **Teen Center,** where specialists in adolescent medicine treat young adult patients in an environment designed for comfort and familiarity. The hospital's comprehensive range of tertiary children's services has made it a referral center for Bangkok and the surrounding areas.

Specialty centers include

✦ **Allergy Clinic:** diagnoses and treats asthma, hay fever, atopic dermatitis, food and drug allergies, and chronic sinusitis.

✦ **Growth, Endocrine, and Diabetes Center for Children:** diagnoses and treats growth hormone deficiency, thyroid disease and abnormalities, precocious and delayed puberty, ambiguous genitalia (including micropenis or undescended testis), adrenal gland disease or disorder, obesity, juvenile diabetes, and other endocrine system disorders.

✦ **Infectious Disease Clinic:** focuses on rare, complicated, or drug-resistant infectious diseases, as well as diagnosis and treatment for all infectious diseases, including bloodstream infections (septicemia), meningitis, pneumonia, and pediatric HIV.

✦ **Pediatric Cardiology Clinic:** offers diagnosis and treatment for congenital heart diseases, abnormal heart rhythm, heart muscle inflammation, pericardial and valve diseases, aortic aneurysm, rheumatic diseases, and Kawasaki disease.

✦ **Pediatric Hearing Center:** conducts complete hearing evaluations and diagnostics, performs cochlear implants, and sells analog and digital hearing aids—much less expensive in Thailand than in the US.

✦ **Pediatric Nephrology Clinic:** provides early detection of kidney disease and abnormalities, as well as treatment for childhood nephrotic syndrome.

✦ **Pediatric Orthopedic Clinic:** focuses on early detection and treatment of bone and joint diseases, as well as treating sports injury, brachial plexus palsy and arm and shoulder paralysis due to difficult delivery, pediatric spinal disorders (such as congenital scoliosis), congenital hip dislocation, and cerebral palsy.

Vejthani Hospital

1 Ladprao Road 111
Khlong-Chan, Bangkapi
Bangkok, THAILAND 10240
Tel: 66 2 734.0000
Fax: 66 2 734.0044
Email: int_mkt@vejthani.com
Web: www.vejthani.com

Established in 1994, Vejthani Hospital was accredited by Thailand's Institute of Hospital Quality Improvement and Accreditation in 2007. Vejthani provides 500 inpatient beds in a 12-story building that also houses 70 clinical examination suites, ten operating theaters, and meeting facilities for 50–80 people—plus a roof garden, restaurants and coffee shops, book and toy shops, and a traditional Thai massage spa. The hospital treats more than 300,000 patients annually, including international patients from 40 countries. Vejthani has 700 full-time employees; more than 250 physicians and dentists are on staff, most of them with international training and certification. The hospital's Web site lists prices for a large number of specific procedures and package services.

Specialties

✦ Abdominal surgery

✦ Colorectal surgery

✦ Dentistry

✦ Gastrointestinal disorders

✦ Hand and shoulder surgery

✦ Health checkups

✦ Infertility (assisted reproductive technology)

✦ Obstetrics and gynecology

✦ Plastic surgery

✦ Skin and laser treatment

✦ Spine surgery

✦ Total joint replacement

✦ Urology

Services Provided for International Patients

✦ Travel arrangements

✦ Accommodations arrangement, including in-house serviced apartment

✦ Airport pickup and dropoff

✦ International Patient Services Counter and Arabic Customer Services Counter

✦ Language interpretation: Arabic, Bengali, English, German, and Japanese

✦ International menu, including *halal* food

✦ Email correspondence

✦ Prayer room

✦ International insurance coordination (see Web site for a long list of partners)

✦ Offices in many countries (see Web site for contact information)

Achievements and Awards

✦ External Quality Assessment in Clinical Chemistry and Clinical Hormones, Mahidol University

✦ National External Quality Assessment in Tumor Markers, Mahidol University

✦ National External Quality Assessment Scheme for HIV Serology

✦ National Proficiency Testing Scheme for Blood Group Serology, Clinical Immunology, Clinical Microscopy, and Hematology, Bureau of Laboratory Quality Standards, Department of Medical Sciences

✦ Quality in Medical Services, Thailand Consumers Choice Awards, 2007

Yanhee International Hospital

454 Charan Sanitwong Road
Bang-O
Bangkok, THAILAND 10700
Tel: 66 2 879.0300
Email: info@yanhee.net; inter_contact@yanhee.net;
info@yanhee.co.th
Web: www.yanhee.net; www.yanhee.co.th

What started out as Yanhee Polyclinic in 1984 is today Yanhee International Hospital, a modern, ten-story building with 400 beds, serving 2,000 outpatients daily. The hospital is expanding rapidly: a 15-story addition opened in 2009, and another new building to house outpatient facilities is scheduled for completion in 2010. Yanhee employs 95 full-time doctors and 120 part-time health professionals, along with 800 nurses and other staff members. Its facilities include an intensive care unit, dialysis unit, nursery, emergency room, laboratory, and 95 examination rooms and delivery rooms.

Among its several specialties, Yanhee is especially well known for plastic surgery and aesthetic treatments. Its **Beauty Center** offers services in dermatology, cosmetic surgery, treatment of varicose veins, and weight control, and encompasses a **Snoring and Voice Change Center, Hair Center,** and **Permanent Cosmetic Tattoo Center** as well. Aesthetic dentistry, laser dentistry, prosthetics, and oral surgery are provided at the hospital's **Dental Center.** Treatments at the **Naturopathic Center** include acupuncture, colonic irrigation, and Thai traditional medicine. Yanhee's Web site lists prices in US dollar amounts for a large number of individual procedures and treatment packages.

Specialty Centers

+ Beauty Center

+ Bone and Joint Reconstructive Center

+ Dental Center

+ Dialysis Center

+ Digestive System Center

+ Ear, Nose, and Throat Center

+ General Medicine Center

+ General Surgery Center

+ Hemorrhoid Center

+ Naturopathic Center

+ Neurology Center

+ Obstetrics and Gynecology Center

+ Ophthalmology Center

+ Pediatric Center

+ Physical Therapy Center

+ Psychiatry Center

+ Urology Center

+ X-ray Center

Bangkok Hospital Phuket

2/1 Hongyok Utis Road
Mueang
Phuket, THAILAND 83000
Tel: 66 76 25.4425
Fax: 66 76 25.4430
Email: info@phukethospital.com
Web: www.phukethospital.com

A sister hospital to Bangkok Hospital Medical Center (described previously), Bangkok Hospital Phuket (BHP) belongs to the Bangkok Hospital Group, a network of 15 private hospitals that collectively forms the largest healthcare provider in Southeast Asia. BHP opened in 1995, and serves both local people and tourists from 127 nationalities who flock to Phuket on vacation. BHP received JCI accreditation in 2009.

The hospital offers a full range of services, including cardiology, cardiothoracic surgery, general surgery, internal medicine, neurology, oncology, orthopedic surgery, radiology, routine health screenings, and urology. Specialties include closed- and open-heart surgery, keyhole surgery, and hip and knee replacement. In 2005 BHP opened its own **International Medical Service Center** catering exclusively to medical travelers. The hospital boasts a full-service dental clinic as well as an **Aesthetic Center** that provides a full range of plastic surgeries (cosmetic and reconstructive). There's an emphasis on prevention at BHP, and several package-priced screening and diagnostic test combinations are listed on the hospital's Web site.

Following extensive damage in the 2004 tsunami, BHP was relocated to a new building. Its facilities can accommodate 1,000 outpatients and provide beds for 200 inpatients. The hospital houses five operating rooms, ten general intensive care beds, and eight cardiac intensive care beds. Sixty full-time specialists, 40 consulting physicians, and 207 nurses make this Phuket's largest medical facility. BHP also runs 11 outreach clinics at various locations around Phuket.

Specialties

✦ Cardiology and cardiothoracic surgery

✦ Dentistry (crown, bridge, porcelain veneer, tooth whitening)

✦ Facial treatment

✦ General surgery

✦ Hair transplantation

✦ Health screening

✦ Internal medicine

✦ Minimally invasive surgery

✦ Neurology

✦ Oncology

✦ Ophthalmology (LASIK surgery, cataract removal)

✦ Orthopedic surgery (hip replacement, knee replacement)

✦ Plastic surgery (breast augmentation, facelift, liposuction, skin and tissue tightening, tummy tuck)

✦ Radiology

✦ Urology

Specialty Centers

✦ Aesthetic Center

✦ Allergy Clinic

✦ Internal Medicine Clinic

✦ Surgery Clinic

Services Provided for International Patients

✦ Language interpretation: English, Filipino, French, German, Italian, Japanese, Russian, and Scandinavian

✦ Assistance with insurance, onward travel arrangements, embassy contact, and repatriation

Achievements and Awards

✦ Superbrands Award Thailand, 2003

✦ Best Service Provider, Prime Minister's Export Award, 2004

✦ Hospital Accreditation, Thailand's Institute of Hospital Quality Improvement and Accreditation, 2004 and 2008

Phuket International Hospital

44 Chalermphrakiet Ro 9 Road
Phuket, THAILAND 83000
Tel: 66 76 24.9400
Fax: 66 76 21.0936
Email: info@phuketinternationalhospital.com
Web: www.phuketinternationalhospital.com

Founded in 1982, Phuket International Hospital (PIH) was the first private hospital to open its doors on the island. Its personnel provide a comprehensive range of general and specialty medical and surgical services, including cardiology, extensive trauma care, hyperbaric treatment for diving emergencies, LASIK eye surgery, neurosurgery, obstetrics, pediatrics, dialysis, and more. PIH is internationally recognized for its plastic surgery. Other specialty areas include orthopedic surgery, dentistry, and general surgery.

PIH was extensively remodeled during 2007, and its new wing contains an outpatient facility and more patient rooms, which have increased the hospital's occupancy to 150 beds. Emergency medical services are provided around the clock seven days a week, and the critical care facilities include 11 intensive care beds.

PIH aggressively promotes its medical checkup packages tailored for Western patients. A variety of tests and exam packages are offered at prices well below fees encountered in the US. For those interested in alternative therapies, the hospital's **Traditional Health Center** offers an array of traditional Chinese medical treatments, including acupuncture, massage, and cupping (the use of suction cups in place of needles at acupuncture points). PIH treats more than 2,000 patients from the US and Canada annually.

Specialties

+ Cardiology
+ Child psychiatry
+ Ear, nose, and throat
+ Emergency medicine
+ General medicine
+ General surgery
+ Hair restoration
+ Health checkups
+ Hyperbaric treatment
+ Obstetrics
+ Pediatrics
+ Plastic surgery
+ Traumatology

Specialty Centers

+ Allergy Clinic
+ Children's Center
+ Dental Center
+ Eye and LASIK Center

+ Hemodialysis Center
+ Lithotripsy Clinic
+ Neurosurgery Clinic
+ Orthopedic Clinic
+ Rheumatology Clinic
+ Skin and Laser Center
+ Traditional Health Center
+ Women's Clinic

Services Provided for International Patients

+ Assistance to patients and referring physicians seeking a consultation, a second opinion, or treatment for a complex illness or injury
+ Appointment scheduling
+ Transportation arrangements, including ground or air ambulance and international medical evacuation
+ Assistance with financial arrangements, including advance estimates for fees, deposits, and payments
+ Coordination of the admission, hospital stay, and discharge process
+ Multilanguage interpretation
+ Coordination of arrangements with third-party insurance companies, embassies, and other businesses

Health Travel Agents
Serving Thailand

BridgeHealth International, Inc.

5299 Denver Tech Center Boulevard, Suite 800
Greenwood Village, CO 80111
Tel: 800 680.1366 (US and Canada toll-free); 303 457.5734
Fax: 303 779.0366
Email: info@bridgehealthintl.com
Web: www.bridgehealthintl.com

In addition to Thailand, BridgeHealth International (BHI) sends patients to Costa Rica, India, Mexico, Singapore, Turkey, and other countries. Serving the business and insurance markets as well as individual consumers, the BHI staff has a lot of experience in steering clients through the medical travel process.

Before accepting a client, BHI screens for health and "travelability." Clients pay no facilitation fees; the fees are paid by the agency's list of approved physicians, clinics, and hospitals (JCI-accredited or equivalent only). Services include passport and visa assistance, airline reservations, medical consultations, medical records transfer assistance, full in-country concierge services, pre-operative and post-operative counseling, and followup care arrangements.

Companion Global Healthcare, Inc.

c/o BlueCross BlueShield of South Carolina
I-20 at Alpine Road, AX-724
Columbia, SC 29219
Tel: 800 906.7065 (US toll-free)
Fax: 803 264.7063
Email: info@companionglobalhealthcare.com
Web: www.companionglobalhealthcare.com

Companion Global Healthcare started out working with hospitals in Ireland and Thailand, and it has since expanded its reach to include Brazil, Costa Rica, Germany, India, Mexico, Singapore, South Korea, Taiwan, and Turkey. In Thailand, this agency sends patients to Bumrungrad International Hospital. Although Companion Global is a wholly owned subsidiary of BlueCross BlueShield of South Carolina, anyone in the US can use its services. At present, followup care upon return from medical travel is provided in South Carolina only, but that situation may change as the agency works with BlueCross BlueShield and other insurance carriers to expand their activities and support of low-cost, fully credentialed medical travel.

Companion Global's Web site offers a click-to-talk capability, and its 24-hour call center offers help to health travelers in a whopping 20 languages! The agency's standard package includes case management, medical record transfer, and travel coordination. Depending on the patient's diagnosis, treatment, and benefit plan, insurance carriers may pay significant portions of the cost. Uninsured customers and clients of other insurance companies pay overseas providers directly. Door-to-door transport, continuing care services, and medical travel insurance cost extra.

This agency estimates big savings when comparing average US southeastern-region prices to Thai prices. For example, a heart bypass costing $144,000 in the southeastern US costs US$23,000–25,000 at Bumrungrad, and a hip replacement priced at US$11,000–14,000 at Bumrungrad averages about $100,000 in the US. Across a number of procedures, Companion Global predicts an average 85 percent savings in medical costs (not including travel expenses).

Cosmetic Surgery Travel, LLC

In the US:
20701 North Scottsdale Road, Suite 107–478
Scottsdale, AZ 85255
Tel: 406 626.5217
Fax: 602 513.7214
Email: medconcierge@cosmeticsurgerytravel.com
Web: www.cosmeticsurgerytravel.com; www.InterMedGlobal.com; www.mtqua.org

In Thailand:
Sukhumvit Soi 63
Ekamai
Bangkok, THAILAND 10110
Tel: 66 85 188.6804

Cosmetic Surgery Travel, in operation since 2002, is the oldest health travel agency in Thailand. It sends Thailand-bound patients to Bumrungrad International Hospital, the Bangkok Hospital Group (including Bangkok International Hospital and Bangkok Heart Hospital at Bangkok Hospital Medical Center), and the Samitivej Group hospitals, working closely with selected surgeons and specialist physicians at its chosen facilities. Originally serving clients who needed multiple plastic surgery procedures—such as body lifts after massive weight loss, or complete face and body makeovers incorporating dental surgery and hair transplantation—the agency now also handles most acute surgery cases, including cardiac, gastric bypass, orthopedic, and refractive and vision surgery, laparoscopic spine surgery, and neurosurgery, as well as stem cell treatment for peripheral artery disease and end-stage heart disease, in vitro fertilization, gynecological disorders, and radiation and chemotherapy treatments.

The agency's founder, Julie Munro, cohosts the world's only medical travel and tourism talk radio show. She also leads the Medical Travel and Tourism Quality Alliance (MTQuA.org), an industry group that promotes safety and medical excellence for traveling patients, encourages professionalism in medical travel and tourism, and raises industry standards. Her agency's services include patient counseling, medical records transfer and review, face-to-face consultation with surgeon(s) prior to surgery, and continuing medical and surgical evaluation and followup. A personal international patient care coordinator arranges and schedules all services and accompanies patients to their appointments. Clients receive kits of wellness and healthcare products and an orchid bouquet on arrival and at discharge.

Healthbase Online, Inc.

287 Auburn Street
Newton, MA 02466
Tel: 888 691.4584 (US and Canada toll-free); 617 418.3436
Fax: 800 986.9230 (US and Canada toll-free)
Email: info.hb@healthbase.com
Web: www.healthbase.com

Healthbase Online, a Boston-based medical tourism facilitator, is organized as a one-stop source for medical travel logistics and concierge services. Healthbase connects patients with internationally accredited (mainly JCI-accredited) hospitals in Belgium, Brazil, Costa Rica, Hungary, India, Malaysia, Mexico, New Zealand, Panama, the Philippines, Singapore, South Korea, Spain, Thailand, Turkey, and the US. In Thailand, it works with Bangkok Hospital Medical Center and Piyavate International Hospital. The agency expects soon to expand its services to Argentina, Australia, Canada, the Czech Republic, El Salvador, Guatemala, Jordan, Poland, South Africa, Taiwan, and the UK.

Healthbase prides itself on exclusive, friendly, and personalized care and round-the-clock customer support. Promising cost savings to organizations and reduced healthcare premiums for clients, the agency serves individual consumers, self-funded businesses, insurers, benefits plan consultants, third-party administrators, and users of consumer-directed healthcare plans or voluntary benefit plans. Healthbase offers customized corporate medical tourism plans for employers and insurance companies. Other services include medical and dental loan financing and travel insurance.

Through the Healthbase online research tool—designated "Best Website for Accessing International Medical Information for Patients/Consumers" in 2007 by *Consumer Health World*—members can explore the medical procedures available and the hospitals offering them, correspond with hospitals and physicians, and share digitized medical records. This secure Web-based system provides instant connectivity with the agency's partner hospitals for speedy, efficient, and effective handling of medical travel inquiries.

International Medical Resources, LLC

9492 Good Lion Road
Columbia, MD 21045
Tel: 410 992.3436
Fax: 410 992.3437
Email: info@medinfoonline.com; jamesperry@medinfoonline.com
Web: www.medinfoonline.com

International Medical Resources (IMR) is a US-based agency that sends patients to Bangkok Hospital Medical Center and to several large hospitals in Singapore. The agency arranges general medical and surgical procedures, cosmetic surgery, and dentistry. IMR founder James Perry says that the medical providers he uses can provide unusual services (for example, intracardiac stem cell therapy and robotic prostate surgery), services typically unavailable in the US (such as Birmingham hip resurfacing), and exceptional quality and personal service.

Unlike staff members in some other health travel firms, Perry and his team have significant medical experience. Perry is a physician associate (PA) with more than 25 years of surgical and medical experience. Although US liability concerns preclude IMR from offering specific medical advice (practicing medicine over the Internet), Perry believes that his medical expertise gives his agency an advantage in communicating with physicians and hospitals and evaluating the quality of services.

Several of this agency's core staff members are Thai, and others have lived and traveled in Thailand, engaging in a wide variety of sport, leisure, and cultural activities. "We are happy to share our local knowledge with clients who are interested," Perry says. For its patients in Thailand, the agency provides an English-speaking guide who accompanies them through the entire treatment process.

Mediseekers

191/1 Soi Chareon Sook
Khlong Toei, Khlong Toei
Bangkok, THAILAND 10110
Tel: 66 2 663.8108
Fax: 66 2 663.8109
Email: info@mediseekers.com
Web: www.mediseekers.com

Mediseekers, established in 2007, specializes in cosmetic and elective surgeries and offers a number of popular packages on its Web site. In Thailand, this agency sends patients to Bangkok Hospital Medical Center, Yanhee International Hospital, and Apex Clinic. Staff members speak English and Thai, as do the doctors who accept Mediseekers patients. Patients in the US enjoy unlimited consultations with a qualified personal manager who helps clients acquire all the knowledge necessary to experience a successful medical retreat. The agency arranges teleconferencing and email exchanges between doctor and patient.

Mediseekers prides itself on its flexibility and can design tailor-made packages to suit any budget. Prospective patients receive a thorough quotation, including pricing, hospital information, doctor's bio and recommendations, and suggested hotel accommodations. Through its affiliation with Expedia, Mediseekers can offer discounted airfares, and booking through the agency's Web site can result in a price break on hotels, too. In Thailand, the patient's personal assistant (for an extra fee) handles transportation arrangements and communications. For those who cannot afford a medical procedure right away, an affiliate of Mediseekers will help locate a finance company to provide a loan, in many cases interest-free for one year to those with good credit ratings.

Med Journeys

120 South Mountain Avenue
Montclair, NJ 07042
Tel: 888 633.5769 (US toll-free); 212 931.0557
Fax: 212 656.1134
Email: mj-info@medjourneys.com
Web: www.medjourneys.com

Med Journeys sends most of its clients to Costa Rica, India, Mexico, and Thailand, but has also cemented relationships with hospitals in other countries. This agency works with Bangkok Hospital Medical Center in Thailand. Since its establishment in

2005, Med Journeys has sent more than 350 patients abroad, and the numbers are growing.

The agency's standard package includes the medical procedure, accommodations during recuperation (including three meals daily), airfare, private transportation in the host country, and premium concierge services. Extra fees are generally charged for optional tours, companions, extended stays, and added medical procedures. Med Journeys encourages clients to contact physicians directly to check references and ask questions about procedures and treatments.

MedRetreat

2042 Laurel Valley Drive
Vernon Hills, IL 60061
Tel: 877 876.3373 (US toll-free); 443 451.9996
Fax: 847 680.0484
Email: customerservice@medretreat.com
Web: www.medretreat.com

In operation since 2003, MedRetreat is one of the better-established US-based health travel agencies, sending patients to Argentina, Brazil, Costa Rica, El Salvador, India, Malaysia, Mexico, South Africa, Thailand, and Turkey. MedRetreat sends Thailand-bound patients to the Phyathai Group hospitals and Piyavate International Hospital. Members receive personalized service through a boutique-style program designed to meet their specific needs. This process includes acquiring hospital information, physicians' credentials, and doctors' consultations; collecting and disseminating medical records; completing price quotations; and arranging procedures, passport and visa acquisition, air travel, travel insurance, financing, destination ground transportation, post-operative hotel booking, and more.

MedRetreat provides 24-hour access to a US program manager, concierge services in the treatment destination, communications while abroad, and assistance once back home. MedRetreat also offers an unconditional money-back guarantee. Its services are free on a first-come, first-served basis.

Planet Hospital

23679 Calabasas Road, Suite 150
Calabasas, CA 91302
Tel: 800 243.0172 (US toll-free); 818 591.1668
Fax: 818 665.4801
Email: rudy@planethospital.com
Web: www.planethospital.com

Rudy Rupak founded Planet Hospital in 2002, after being impressed with the quality of care his fiancée received when she fell ill in Thailand, and the agency has since sent more than 3,000 patients abroad for medical care. It currently serves Argentina, Belgium, Brazil, Costa Rica, Cyprus, Dubai, El Salvador, India, Malaysia, Malta, Mexico, Panama, the Philippines, Singapore, South Korea, Thailand, Turkey, and the US. Planet Hospital sends Thailand-bound patients to Bumrungrad International Hospital, the Samitivej Group of hospitals, Piyavate International Hospital, Yanhee International Hospital, Preecha Aesthetic Institute (cosmetic surgery), LasikThai (LASIK eye surgery), and Promjai Dental. The agency's in-country concierges take care of clients from the moment they land to the moment they leave, and its representatives personally inspect every hospital and doctor the agency recommends.

Planet Hospital currently works with several self-insured employers who have contracted its services to help their employees save money. Specialties include cardiovascular procedures, cosmetic surgery, dentistry, fertility/reproduction (including surrogacy), oncology, and orthopedics. Planet Hospital is the only medical travel agency that has been a member of the Better Business Bureau since 2002 with an AA rating.

The agency's Web site offers a comprehensive list of major hospitals in its service areas, along with a sampling of its top recommended physicians. Planet Hospital requires its physicians to pass a certification exam from the American Board of Quality Assurance and Utilization Review Physicians (ABQAURP), the US's largest organization of interdisciplinary healthcare professionals.

Satori World Medical

591 Camino De La Reina, Suite 407
San Diego, CA 92108
Tel: 619 704.2000
Fax: 619 704.2049
Email: j.yarbrough@satoriworldmedical.com
Web: www.satoriworldmedical.com

Satori World Medical started operating in 2007, and its growing network includes hospitals in Costa Rica, India, Mexico, the Philippines, Singapore, Thailand, and Turkey. The agency sends Thailand-bound patients to Bangkok Hospital Medical Center, Bumrungrad International Hospital, and Preecha Aesthetic Institute. Its clients include self-funded employers, health plans, unions, trusts, municipalities, third-party administrators, benefit brokers, and consultants. Satori's staff members speak English, Spanish, Japanese, and Farsi.

Satori's patient advocates are nurses who coordinate all inquiries, from discussing procedures with the patient and facilitating medical records transfer to scheduling followup care and educating companions on their responsibilities. The agency's travel care coordinators schedule procedure dates with the hospital, make airline and hotel reservations, coordinate ground transportation, and provide 24-hour customer service. Package pricing includes all procedure, hospital, and physician fees; roundtrip airfare for the patient and a companion; a two-week stay at an Intercontinental hotel; and a personal accident insurance policy.

SOS Medical Tourism Services Co., Ltd.

6/36 Wiset Road
Fisherman's Way, Rawai
Phuket, THAILAND 83100
Tel: 66 86 973.8074
Email: sosmedical@ymail.com
Web: www.sosmedicaltourism.net

This agency, founded in 2008, serves clients from Australia, Denmark, France, Germany, Japan, the Netherlands, New Zealand, Sweden, and the US. It sends about 10–15 patients each month to the Bangkok Hospital Group, Piyavate International Hospital, Phuket International Hospital, Jungceylon Plastic Surgery Clinic, Phuket Aesthetics Surgery Clinic, Bangkok Dental Smile, Phuket SEA Smile Clinic, Atmanjai Detox Center, and more. Staff members speak English, French, Japanese, German, and Thai.

SOS arranges cosmetic and reconstructive surgeries, knee and hip surgery, eye surgery (LASIK), dental treatments and implants, sex reassignment and facial feminization procedures, and alternative health treatments, such as body detoxification, yoga, medical spa stays, and acupuncture treatments. The agency assists with visa and visa extensions, online medical correspondence, appointment scheduling, airline and hotel bookings, airport transportation, hospital admissions, and followup care back home. An SOS case manager visits hospital inpatients daily.

ThaiMed International, Ltd.

#2C 24 Sukhumvit Soi 11
Khlong Toei
Bangkok, THAILAND 10110
Tel: 888 THAI.MED (842.4633) (US toll-free); 66 2 195.5130
Fax: 66 2 195.5131
Email: contact@thaimed.us
Web: www.thaimakeover.com

ThaiMed International, which specializes in cosmetic surgery, was established after its CEO and founder, Mike Brennan—then a self-employed, uninsured American living in Japan—sought aesthetic procedures for himself in Thailand. Having "learned the ropes" through experience, he now provides the service he wishes he had received when he was a medical traveler. On the agency's Web site, Brennan displays his own photographs before and after hair transplant, upper and lower eyelid lifts, facial filler, liposuction, and dermatological treatments.

Brennan prides himself on individualizing plans to meet each client's unique needs. "A week or a month, five-star to budget, everything is flexible and entirely up to you," he says. ThaiMed provides airport pickup and all transfers to and from the hotel, hospital, and medical appointments, as well as a personal assistant who helps with everything from shopping and sightseeing to followup on doctors' visits. The agency also arranges loans and finance plans for US patients who undergo orthopedic, plastic, or bariatric (weight loss) surgery, heart procedures, and kidney transplantation in Thailand.

ThaiMed's surgical and medical patients go to Bumrungrad International Hospital, Piyavate International Hospital, Bangkok Hospital Medical Center, Vichaiyut Hospital, Bangkok Nursing Home Hospital, Saint Louis Hospital, the Samitivej Group of hospitals, Yanhee International Hospital, and Praram 9 Hospital. Dental patients go to Bangkok Smile Dental Clinic and Dental Hospital. Eye patients go to TRSC LASIK Eye Center, Rutnin Eye Hospital, and Laser Vision Eye Clinic. Some cosmetic and restorative procedures are arranged at the Skin and Allergy Clinic and Stough Hair Clinic.

Wellness Travel Company, Ltd.

Villa Wellness 7/1
Sukhumvit Soi 14
Bangkok, THAILAND 10110
Tel: 66 2 229.4862
Fax: 66 2 229.5188
Email: customercare@wellnesstravel.com;
enquiries@wellnesstravel.com
Web: www.wellnesstravel.com

Wellness Travel Company serves Thailand, Singapore, Malaysia, and India. Since 2004 it has been sending patients to Thailand's Piyavate International Hospital and Yanhee International Hospital. Clients can purchase a membership card called a MyWellcard that entitles them to specially priced, all-inclusive medical and surgical treatment packages, covering all fees and necessary inclusions for a standard surgery. According to the agency, using the card significantly reduces healthcare, travel, and medical costs for individuals and families. Airport transportation, hotel accommodation, and all medical costs are covered in the package price. Wellness Travel offers complimentary upgrades of hotel and hospital rooms, complimentary in-room Internet service, airport transfer with private vehicle and chauffeur, assistance with visa extensions, assistance with day-trips and shopping excursions, and translation services. The agency's Web site presents several testimonials from satisfied customers.

PART THREE

Spa Destinations in the Land of Smiles

For tired, stressed, worried medical travelers who need to unwind before undergoing some medical procedure—or for those who'd like to recover in a tranquil environment complete with a bit of pampering—the spas of Thailand are the perfect destination. And the spa experience may do more than rest your mind and body; it may actually promote your healing process. Part Three features a wide variety of tempting Thai spas.

Introduction

Spa-going, wellness, and relaxation are a way of life in Thailand, so no matter where you travel, you'll find a spa nearby. If you have only an afternoon to spare, you can easily stop by a convenient facility for a vigorous traditional Thai massage or a more gentle oil massage. But if your schedule, budget, and medical condition permit, you may want to set aside a week or two for an indulgent, rejuvenating vacation at a resort spa.

Incorporating elements of Indian Ayurvedic medicine and Chinese medicine, the core philosophies of traditional Thai therapies revolve around the balance of the four basic elements— earth, water, wind, and fire—which constitute the essence of life and appear as recurrent themes in many modern spas. Thai massage techniques were originally introduced by a traveling Indian doctor and have been passed down from teacher to student since the second or third century, when they were first practiced at Bangkok's Wat Pho, "the Temple of the Reclining Buddha." The traditional Thai massage, often utilizing an herbal ball, is a memorable experience. In this oil-free massage, the therapist applies a sometimes strenuous combination of pressure, pulling, and stretching to correct energy imbalances, stimulate the flow of *prana* (breath or life energy), and restore general well-being.

Thailand attracts spa-goers from all over the world with the abundance and diversity of its approaches and treatments. Nearly every kind of spa service can be found in Thailand: traditional Thai massage, oil massage, hot stone massage, reflexology, fragrant herbal compresses and steams, scrubs, wraps, facials, bath soaks, floats, detox programs, rejuvenation programs, weight loss programs, yoga, tai chi, meditation, and more. As most medical travelers never get out of Bangkok, we feature mostly city spas here, but we also include a few outside Bangkok and three additional spas on the island of Phuket.

Some Spas in Thailand

IN BANGKOK

Ananda Spa

(At the Capitol Club)
99397 Sukhumvit 24
Khlongton, Khlong Toei
Bangkok, THAILAND 10110
Tel: 66 2 661.1210
Fax: 66 2 261.2145
Email: spamgr@thecapitolclub.com
Web: www.thecapitolclub.com; www.anandaspa.net

Located in the heart of Bangkok in the shopping hub at Sukhumvit is the Capitol Club, where a 33-foot (10-meter) rock-climbing wall takes center stage, with two overlooking levels of state-of-the-art cardiovascular exercise equipment. The facility houses tennis and squash courts, swimming pools, Jacuzzis, food and beverage outlets, and the world-class Ananda Spa.

The spa's name is derived from the Sanskrit word for harmony, and the name is apt. Ananda's staff members use holistic massage and aromatherapy to rejuvenate the body and uplift the spirit. Options available to guests include massages, scrubs, baths, hair treatments, and traditional Thai massage. On offer are tailor-made spa packages, including one for men and another for couples. Special spa services and prices are available to Capitol Club members and walk-in clients.

Additional Locations in Thailand

Another one in Bangkok:

> Ananda Spa
> (At the President Solitaire)
> Sukhumvit Soi 11
> Bangkok, THAILAND 10110
> Tel: 66 2 255.7200
> Fax: 66 2 253.2330

Type: Day

Signature Services

✦ Ananda Facial

✦ Ananda Hot Stone Massage

✦ Ananda Jet Lag Energizer (body massage with aromatherapy oil, head massage, and a cup of tea)

✦ Ananda Spa Massage

✦ Ananda Spa Retreat (herbal body polish, massage, and facial)

Cost: Massages and facials start at 1,500 baht (about US$44). The Ananda Spa Retreat package costs 3,795 baht (about US$112).

Spa Cenvaree

(At Centara Grand at CentralWorld)
999/99 Rama 1 Road
Pathumwan
Bangkok, THAILAND 10330
Tel: 66 2 100.1234
Fax: 66 2 100.1235
Email: spacenvareecgcw@chr.co.th
Web: www.spacenvaree.com

Spa Cenvaree's caregivers believe all ailments originate from an imbalance among the three pillars of well-being: body, mind, and soul. Spa treatments here promote the holistic theme of achieving balance in life by treating the three pillars as one. Citing water as the source of life, Cenvaree's spa treatments complement the healing powers of water with the curative powers of Thai herbs, flower essences, aromatherapy, and human touch. Services include massage, body polish, body wrap, facials, and nail care, plus treatments and packages specially tailored for men. Cenvaree is part of the Centara group, which operates hotels and resorts in Bangkok, Chiang Mai, Hat Yai, Hua Hin, Phangan, Krabi, Mae Sot, Pattaya, Phuket, Samui, Trat, Udon Thani, and the Maldives.

Additional Locations in Thailand

Twelve other locations, including this one in Bangkok:

Spa Cenvaree
(At Sofitel Centara Grand Bangkok)
1695 Phaholyothin Road
Chatuchak
Bangkok, THAILAND 10900
Tel: 66 2 541.1234
Fax: 66 2 541.1087
Email: spacenvareescgb@chr.co.th

Type: Day

Signature Services

✤ Cenvaree Pa-Lang Experience (massage using heated Himalayan river stones coated with warm oils)

✤ Malako Quenching Body Care (fresh papaya body brush and warm, aromatic oil body wrap)

✤ Vitalizer Men's Package (traditional Thai massage, with choice of scalp or foot massage)

Awards

✤ Asia's Best New Spa, Asia Spa & Wellness Festival, 2009

✤ Thailand Gold Spa Award, Ministry of Public Health, 2009

Cost: The Cenvaree Pa-Lang Experience costs 2,895 baht (about US$84). The Vitalizer Men's Package is priced at 3,500 baht (about US$103).

Devarana Spa

(At Dusit Thani Bangkok)
946 Rama IV Road
Silom, Bangrak
Bangkok, THAILAND 10500
Tel: 66 2 636.3596; 66 2 200.9000
Fax: 66 2 636.3597
Email: bangkok@devaranaspa.com
Web: www.devaranaspa.com

Conveniently situated near a subway stop and a Bangkok Transit System (BTS) Sky Train station, Devarana Spa at Bangkok's Dusit Thani Hotel is an oasis of tranquility in the heart of Thailand's bustling capital. The word *devarana* (pronounced tee-WAH-run) means "garden in heaven" in Sanskrit, and the name is apt. Devarana's designers set out to recreate a heavenly garden to pamper guests in a soothing, stress-relieving environment.

Devarana Spa offers services at select five-star hotels—four in Thailand and two in Italy and the Philippines. Each one emphasizes East-meets-West health and beauty practices derived from age-old therapies and updated with a modern twist. On the menu are massages, body scrubs and wraps, facials, water treatments, and a variety of specialized packages.

Additional Locations in Thailand

Three other locations, including this one in Hua Hin:

Devarana Spa
(At Dusit Thani Hua Hin)
1349 Phetchakasem Road
Cha-Am Phetchaburi
Hua Hin, THAILAND 76120
Tel: 66 32 44.2494
Fax: 66 32 44.2495
Email: huahin@devaranaspa.com

Type: Resort/hotel

Treatment Rooms: Nine standard rooms, four deluxe suites for two people, one grand suite for two people

Signature Services

✦ Devarana Bath

✦ Devarana Body Scrub

✦ Devarana Massage

✦ Devarana Touch of Heaven (60- or 90-minute facial and 90-minute body massage)

Awards

✦ Best Scrub, *SpaAsia* Crystal Awards, 2004

✦ Favorite Spa, *Bangkok Magazine* Readers Choice Awards, 2006–2007

✦ Best Urban Spa, *Anywhere* Travel Awards, 2007

✦ Best Urban Spa, *Lifestyle and Travel* Readers Choice Awards, 2008

✦ Best Spa, *Living in Thailand* Awards, 2008

Cost: The Devarana Bath costs 990 baht (about US$30). The price range for Devarana Touch of Heaven packages is 4,900–6,000 baht (about US$144–176).

Health Land Spa & Massage Sathon

120 North Sathon Road
Silom, Bangrak
Bangkok, THAILAND 10500
Tel: 66 2 637.8883
Fax: 66 2 634.5353
Email: info@healthlandspa.com
Web: www.healthlandspa.com

Health Land Spa & Massage originally began as a health complex comprising a supermarket of organic and health foods, vegetarian restaurant, drugstore, herb garden, library, massage and meditation room, and a seminar corner for those who wanted to discuss health matters. This complex was later transformed into a complete spa service center. Srinakarin was the first branch, followed by Sathon, Pinklao, Pattaya, and Ekamai.

All Health Land locations are stand-alone structures with convenient access and spacious parking lots. And while its facilities are luxurious, Health Land boasts prices that are generally lower than those charged by hotel-based spas. Its customers include expatriates, office workers, housewives, and university students, as well as foreign customers who travel from overseas.

Additional Locations in Thailand

Four other locations, including these three in Bangkok:

Health Land Srinakarin
7021 Mu 2
Srinakarin Road
Nongbon, Phawet
Bangkok, THAILAND 10260
Tel: 66 2 748.8135
Fax: 66 2 746.5376

Health Land Pinklao
1426 Charan Sanitwong Road
Arun Amarin, Bangkok Noi
Bangkok, THAILAND 10700
Tel: 66 2 882.4888
Fax: 66 2 882.4612

Health Land Ekamai
961 Soi Sukhumvit 63
Sukhumvit Road, Ekamai
Phra Khanong Nua, Wattana
Bangkok, THAILAND 10110
Tel: 66 2 392.2233
Fax: 66 2 392.2234

Type: Day

Signature Services

✦ Aromatherapy Body Massage

✦ Body Polish

✦ Traditional Thai Massage

Cost: The Traditional Thai Massage is a bargain at about 450 baht (about US$13); so is the Aromatherapy Body Massage at 850 baht (about US$25).

Leela Thai Herbal Spa, Sathon Branch

43 Soi Narathiwat 7
Sathon
Bangkok, THAILAND 10120
Tel: 66 2 679.3511
Email: contact@leelathaispa.com
Web: www.leelathaispa.com

Leela Thai Herbal Spa's flagship operation on Soi Thonglo has now expanded to this second location, offering a range of massage therapies, spa treatments, Dead Sea treatments by Paloma, and facial treatments by Guinot. The atmosphere is a mixture of exotic Asia with a touch of lemongrass-scented contemporary. Traditional Thai herbal treatments are available, as are relaxing aromatherapy massages. Leela masseuses can blend both techniques together in one session for maximum results. A complimentary footbath and a cup of warm bael fruit tea (*nam matum* in Thai) are given to each guest before every treatment.

Additional Locations in Thailand

The original, also in Bangkok:

> Leela Thai Herbal Spa, Thonglo Branch
> 4404 Opposite Soi Thonglo 15
> Sukhumvit 55
> Bangkok, THAILAND 10110
> Tel: 66 2 714.8500

Type: Day

Treatment Rooms: Two steam rooms, two couple massage rooms (one with Jacuzzi), 11 single massage rooms, four seats for foot massage

Signature Services

✦ Dead Sea Exotic (body scrub, black mud wrap, body massage, and lavender-scented bath)

✦ Exotic of Leela Thai (full-body scrub, massage, and bath)

✦ Leela Thai Aroma Massage (traditional Thai massage using a unique blend of essential oils)

✦ Leela Thai Healing Touch (massage for relieving headaches and back pain)

Cost: A Leela Thai Aroma Massage runs about 1,500 baht (about US$44). The Dead Sea Exotic costs 3,200 baht (about US$94).

The Royal Orchid Mandara Spa

(At the Royal Orchid Sheraton Hotel & Towers)
2 Captain Bush Lane
New Road, Siphaya
Bangkok, THAILAND 10500
Tel: 66 2 266.0123
Fax: 66 2 639.5478
Email: ms_shro@minornet.com
Web: www.mandaraspa.com

The name Mandara comes from an ancient Sanskrit legend about the gods' quest to find the elixir of immortality and eternal youth, and many of the spa's signature treatments spring from such Balinese roots. Worldwide, Mandara Spas offer 300 different treatments, with the menu at each spa tailored to that location's theme, design, and clientele. Choices for clients at the Royal Orchid Mandara Spa include Balinese favorites, classic techniques originating from Europe or other parts of Asia, and uniquely Thai offerings.

Located on the third floor of a Sheraton hotel that is one of Bangkok's finest, Mandara's suites feature some of Bangkok's best views of the Chao Phraya River (River of Kings). Facilities include a private plunge pool, steam shower room, and changing room. A full range of face, body, and massage treatments is on offer, including manicures and pedicures, Ayurvedic treatments, and salon services. Full-day, half-day, and couples packages are available, and poolside massages can be arranged.

Additional Locations in Thailand

Five other locations, including these three in Bangkok, Hua Hin, and Phuket:

Mandara Spa
(At Bangkok Marriott Resort & Spa)
2571-3 Charoen Nakhon Road
Krungthep Bridge
Bangkok, THAILAND 10600
Tel: 66 2 476.0021
Fax: 66 2 476.1120

Mandara Spa
(At Hua Hin Marriott Resort & Spa)
1071 Phetchakasem Beach Road
Hua Hin, THAILAND 77110
Tel: 66 32 51.1882
Fax: 66 32 51.2422

Mandara Spa
(At JW Marriott Phuket Resort & Spa)
231 Mu 3
Mai Khao, Thalang
Phuket, THAILAND 83110
Tel: 66 76 33.8000
Fax: 66 76 34.8349

Type: Hotel/resort

Treatment Rooms: Five double rooms, three spa suites, one deluxe suite with an enclosed rooftop garden

Signature Services

✦ Dead Sea Salt Scrub (massage with a mixture of water, salt crystals, and essential oils)

✦ Mandara Massage (two therapists employ Japanese shiatsu, traditional Thai, Hawaiian lomi lomi, Swedish, and Balinese massage techniques)

✦ Shirodhara (massage, Ayurvedic oil flow treatment, scalp massage, and shampoo)

Cost: The Mandara Massage runs about 4,000 baht (about US $118). The Dead Sea Salt Scrub costs 2,000 baht (about US$59).

Oasis Spa Bangkok

64 Soi Sawasdee
Sukhumvit 31 Road
Phra Khanong
Bangkok, THAILAND 10110
Tel: 66 2 262.2122
Email: sales@chiangmaioasis.com
Web: www.bangkokoasis.com

If you yearn for a waterfall in your treatment room, then Oasis Spa Bangkok is for you. Oasis Spas utilize numerous combinations of traditional Thai herbals, each preparation formulated fresh daily. Guests choose from a complete menu of treatments and therapies: scrubs, wraps, Jacuzzi baths, steam baths, massages of the face, feet, and hands, and more. Private spa suites have terraces, Jacuzzis, glass-enclosed steam rooms, outdoor showers, and restrooms. The customer relations specialists here speak five languages. Something you won't find in every spa is the Golden Lanna massage with gold-infused oil offered at Oasis—gold, it's claimed, rebalances the skin and restores aging skin at the cellular level.

Additional Locations in Thailand

Three other locations, including this one in Phuket:

Oasis Spa Phuket
47 Mu 1
Srisunthorn Road
Cherngtalay, Thalang
Phuket, THAILAND 83110
Tel: 66 76 27.0271

Type: Day

Treatment Rooms: Fifteen rooms, with a total capacity for 30 clients

Signature Services

✦ Aroma Hot Oil Massage (Swedish-style massage)

✦ Golden Lanna (gold-infused oil massage)

✦ King of Oasis (massage with herbal hot compresses and hot oil)

✦ Oasis Four Hands Massage (two therapists massage simultaneously)

✦ Queen of Oasis (hot oil aromatherapy massage)

Awards

✦ Most Recognized Service, Prime Minister's Export Award, 2007

✦ Thailand's Most Outstanding Brand, SME Best Brand Award, 2007

✦ Excellent Day Spa, Thailand Tourism Award, 2008

✦ Thai World-Class Spa Certification (one of only 23), Ministry of Public Health, 2009

Cost: The two-hour King of Oasis costs 3,900 baht (about US$115). The Swedish-style Aroma Hot Oil Massage is a bargain at 1,350 baht (about US$40). A 90-minute Golden Lanna massage costs 5,900 baht (about US$174).

Oriental Spa

(At the Mandarin Oriental Hotel)
48 Oriental Avenue
Bangkok, THAILAND 10500
Tel: 66 2 659.9000, ext. 7440
Fax: 66 2 659.9284
Email: mobkk-spa@mohg.com
Web: www.mandarinoriental.com/bangkok/spa

The Mandarin Oriental Hotel has served as a home away from home for such notables as Elizabeth Taylor, Goldie Hawn, and former US president George H. W. Bush. You may not bump into a celebrity at the hotel's Oriental Spa, but you can't miss finding something you like among the many available body treatments, luxurious massages, baths, and facials. Ancient Ayurvedic remedies and aromatherapies are employed. Half-day, full-day, three-day, and week-long packages are offered.

Located in a Thai-style golden teakwood house just across the river from the hotel, the spa recently underwent a renovation to the tune of US$1.2 million. Each treatment room has a private shower, steam room, and tropical-rain-effect showerheads. Some also have Jacuzzi whirlpools and saunas. Other facilities include heated scrub tables, whirlpools, herbal steam bath, *rhassoul* bath (*rhassoul* is a Moroccan clay used to massage the skin), and private manicure and pedicure areas.

Type: Hotel/resort

Treatment Rooms: Fourteen suites

Signature Services

✦ Oriental Body Glow

✦ Oriental Body Wellness

✦ Oriental Luxury Manicure

✦ Oriental Signature Massage

Awards

✦ Best Spa in a Hotel Resort Worldwide, *Gallivanter's Guide for Excellence*, 2005–2006

✦ Best Spa in the World, *Robb Report: World's Best 30th Anniversary Issue*, 2006

✦ Second Place, Top 10 Hotel Spas in the Asia-Pacific, Africa, and Middle East, *Travel+Leisure* World's Best Awards, 2007

✦ Spa's Therapist Team of the Year, *AsiaSpa* Awards, 2007

✦ Best City Spa in the Asia Pacific, *DestinAsian* Readers Choice Awards, 2008

✦ Urban Spa of the Year, *AsiaSpa* Awards, 2008

✦ Twelfth Place, Top 20 Hotel Spas, *Travel+Leisure* World's Best Awards, 2008

Cost: The Oriental Luxury Manicure costs 2,400 baht (about US$70). The price range for massages is 3,500–4,300 baht (US$103–126).

Palm Herbal Retreat

5222 Soi Thonglo 16
Sukhumvit 55 Road
Khlongton Nua, Wattana
Bangkok, THAILAND 10110
Tel: 66 2 391.3254
Fax: 66 2 391.1228
Email: info@palmherbalspa.co.th
Web: www.palmherbalspa.co.th

Located in the heart of Bangkok with easy access via Sky Train (Thonglo Station), Palm Herbal Retreat emphasizes traditional Thai treatments and a homey, unpretentious environment. In addition to conventional massage therapies, Palm offers scrubs, body wraps, baths, facials, fresh herbal packs, aromatherapy, traditional Thai massage, detoxification treatments, paraffin treatments, waxing, and a special postnatal treatment for new moms. Natural Thai herbs are incorporated into the spa treatments with home-brewed herbal tea, freshly made herbal healing compresses, and an herbal-scented steam room. Half-day and full-day packages are available.

Type: Day

Signature Services

✦ Half-Day Spa Body Pamper: Secret of Palm (shower, body wrap, and traditional Thai massage with optional oil)

✦ Massage-Lover Package: The Best of Palm (oil massage, herbal foot massage, and herbal bath)

Cost: The Secret of Palm costs 3,450 baht (about US$101) and the Best of Palm is 2,850 baht (about US$84).

Pranali Wellness Spa, Shinawatra Branch

Shinawatra Tower III, 32nd Floor
1010 Vibhavadi-Rangsit Road
Latyao, Chatuchak
Bangkok, THAILAND 10900
Tel: 66 2 949.2400–2404
Fax: 66 2 949.2405
Web: www.pranaliwellness.com

Pranali Wellness Spa is a health club and spa under one roof. An investment of more than 60 million baht (about US$1.8 million) equipped Pranali with steam rooms, a lounge for relaxing, Internet service, a hair salon, and a spa cuisine and juice bar. Services are offered in slimming, fitness, aesthetics, holistic healing therapies, antiaging, eye and skin management, detoxification, yoga, Pilates, and more. State-of-the-art equipment includes

✦ an Aqua Spa, a professional detoxification system that bathes the feet in ionized water

✦ a Slim-Fit stepper, which incorporates infrared technology to burn more fat than ordinary steppers

✦ a Huber machine, an innovation in exercise equipment that strengthens the back, increases flexibility, and improves coordination

The name Pranali comes from two words: *prana* meaning "breath" and *leela* meaning "rhythm." Breathing is a sign of the life force within, say Pranali staff, and controlling its rhythm promotes maximal physical and mental health. To tailor their products to individual needs, Pranali offers a personalized service called *L'atelier du Pranali*. The service formulates compounds ranging from natural perfume to body cleansers, each customized to the client's personality and lifestyle.

Additional Locations in Thailand

Another one in Bangkok:

Pranali Wellness Spa, Siam Paragon Branch
989 Siam Paragon Tower, 3rd Floor, Unit 334
Rama 1 Road
Pathumwan
Bangkok, THAILAND 10330
Tel: 66 2 610.9596
Fax: 66 2 610.9598

Type: Day

Signature Services

✦ Pranali Detoxifying Treatment Facial

✦ Pranali Marvelous Herbal Compress

✦ Pranali Massage

Treatment Rooms: Ten single rooms, two twin rooms, two hydrotherapy rooms, two traditional Thai massage rooms, two slim-fit rooms, two consultation rooms, one medical assistance room

Award

✦ 150 World-Class Spas, *SpaAsia* Crystal Awards, 2006

Cost: The Pranali Detoxifying Treatment Facial is priced at 1,900 baht (about US$56). Massages are in the range of 1,900–2,500 baht (about US$56–73).

S Medical Spa

2/2 Bhakdi Building
Wireless Road
Lumphini
Bangkok, THAILAND 10330
Tel: 66 2 253.1010
Fax: 66 2 253.9625
Email: info@smedspa.com
Web: www.smedspa.com

S Medical Spa is located in the heart of Bangkok's central business district, a few minutes' walk from the Sky Train Phloenchit Station. The staff of dermatologists, gynecologists, psychiatrists, and spa specialists offers a combination of Western medicine and Eastern therapies, including therapeutic massage, body and facial treatments, holistic body works, antiaging regimens, and purification programs. Several dermatologists oversee skin treatments ranging from vitamin-enriched facials to laser treatments for tightening loose skin in the abdomen and underarms, removing moles, banishing stretch marks, fading age spots, and more.

The two-floor, 29,060-square-foot (2,700-square-meter) facility houses herbal steam rooms, Jacuzzis, a sauna, therapeutic pool, gym, physical assessment room, relaxation lounge, and a spa restaurant. The spa's Medical Department has a pharmacy and a laboratory. S Medical offers its own line of beauty products, from liquid soap to sunscreen to Botox eye gel. Staff members even teach cooking classes.

Type: Day

Treatment Rooms: Twelve spa rooms, two Thai massage rooms, one hydrotherapy room, three purification rooms; in the Medical Department, five consultation rooms, four medical facial rooms, four laser rooms, two body contour rooms, two therapeutic massage rooms, seven spa suites

Signature Services

✦ Carboxy (carbon dioxide infiltration to improve the appearance of cellulite)

✦ Laser Skin Resurfacing

Awards

✦ Medi-Spa of the Year, *AsiaSpa* Awards, 2007

✦ Outstanding Performance, Health Tourism–Oriented Medical Establishment, Tourism Authority of Thailand (TAT) Awards, 2008

✦ Award of Excellence, Medically Oriented Establishment, Thailand Tourism Awards, 2008

Cost: A 90-minute massage and facial costs 6,356 baht (about US$187). You can get a two-hour purification and facial for 9,181 baht (about US$297).

Seven Eden Spa

(At Siri Sathon)
27 Soi Saladaeng 1
Silom Road, Bangrak
Bangkok, THAILAND 10500
Tel: 66 2 266.2345, ext. 49
Fax: 66 2 267.5555
Email: reservation@sirisathorn.com
Web: www.sirisathorn.com

Siri Sathon, a luxury boutique-serviced residence, lies in the heart of Bangkok, with convenient access to the BTS Sky Train. Seven Eden Spa and a fitness club are located on the second floor. Seven Eden's wide range of spa treatments emphasizes natural plant essences and aromatic oils while blending traditional approaches and contemporary practices. Massage offerings include hot stone massage, detoxifying hot clay massage, traditional Thai massage, and aromatherapy balance/renewal massage, along with packages specifically designed for relaxation, rejuvenation, and recovery. Personal trainers and exercise classes are available at the fitness club, and the Siri Sathon Liquid Bar and Café serves light, low-fat, low-calorie meals.

Type: Hotel/resort

Treatment Rooms: One couple room, one couple room with steam room, one couple room for Thai massage, one single room for facial treatment

Signature Services

✦ Anti-Cellulite Wrap

✦ Enliven for Men

✦ Indonesian Lymphatic Massage

✦ Seven Eden Signature Massage

Cost: The Indonesian Lymphatic Massage price range is 1,450–1,750 baht (about US$43–51). The Anti-Cellulite Wrap costs 2,150 baht (about US$63). Enliven for Men is 1,450 baht (about US$43).

Take Care Beauty Salon & Spa

Take Care operates a chain of salons and spas in Bangkok. One branch is a salon only, and one is a nail boutique, but these three provide spa services:

Take Care Beauty Salon & Spa

1216 Sukhumvit 33
Bangkok, THAILAND 10110
Tel: 66 2 662.0805
Email: info@takecarebeauty.com
Web: www.takecarebeauty.com

Take Care Beauty Salon & Spa

Market Place
Sukhumvit 55, 2nd Floor (Soi Thonglo)
Bangkok, THAILAND 10110
Tel: 66 2 392.9690

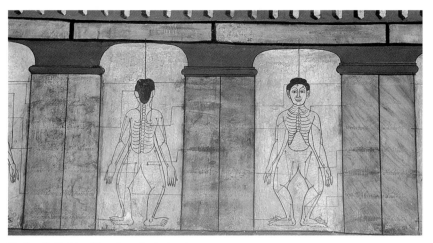

Thailand's first traditional medical school

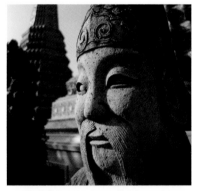

Over 1,000 sculptures and Buddha images

Wat Pho is the oldest and largest Buddhist temple in Bangkok.

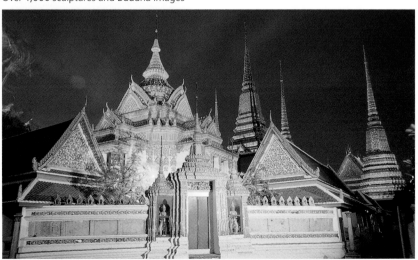

Wat Pho, Temple of the Reclining Buddha

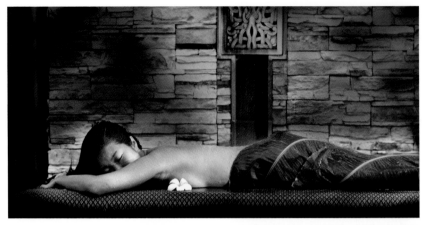

Banyan Tree Spa Rainmist Steam Bath

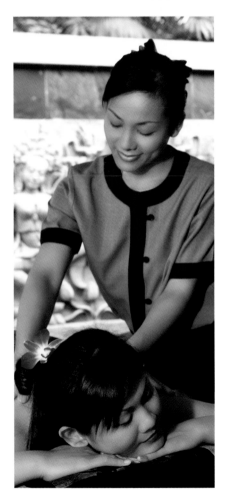

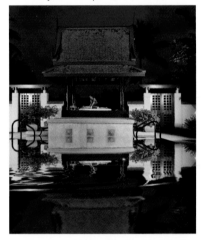

Massage at Sala Spa

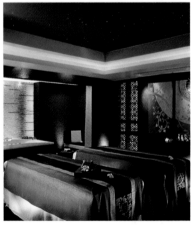

Luxurious Thai massage experience

Grand spa suite

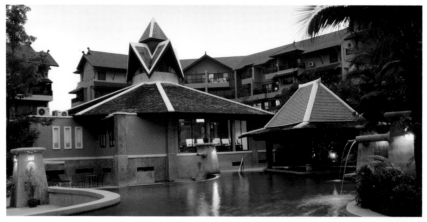

Pattaya Oasis Spa

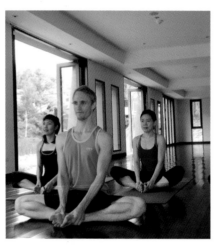

Sukko Spa Ashtanga Yoga Class

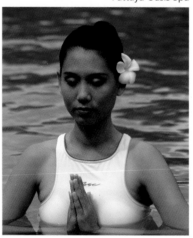

Sukko Spa Aqua Exercise

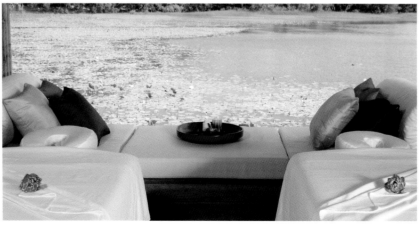

Oasis Secret Garden Spa

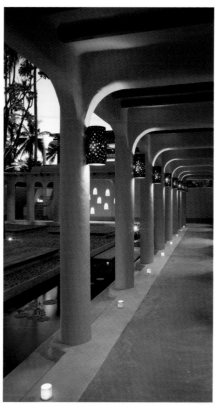

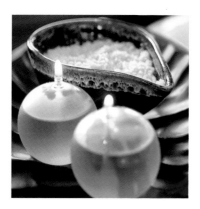

Pamper
yourself in
one of
Thailand's
many spas.

One of Thailand's many elegant spa retreats

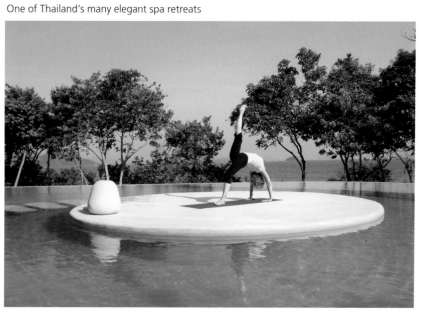

Thailand is a leading destination for yoga

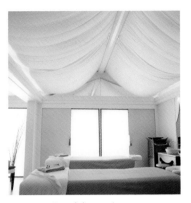

Devarana Spa deluxe suite

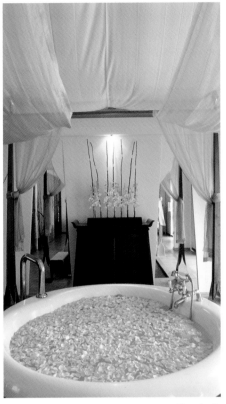

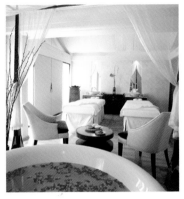

In-suite floral bath

Devarana Spa yellow bath

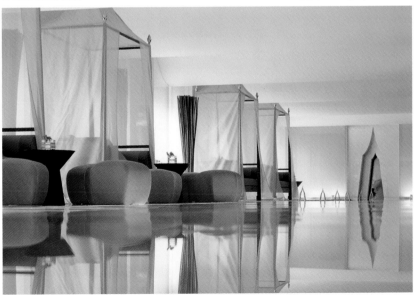

Devarana Spa lobby

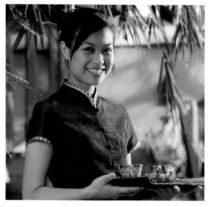

A friendly welcome

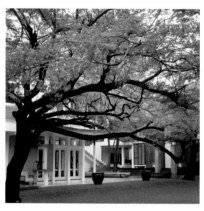

Bangkok Oasis Spa

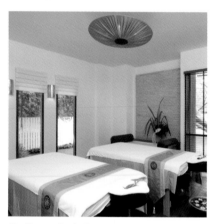

Healing and relaxing treatment room

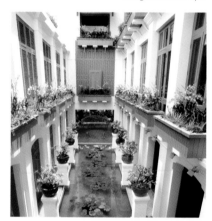

Mandarin Oriental Spa

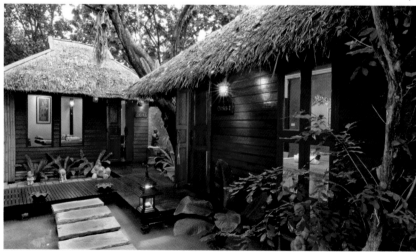

Chiangmai Oasis Spa

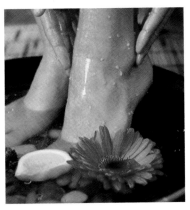
Soothing foot-soak

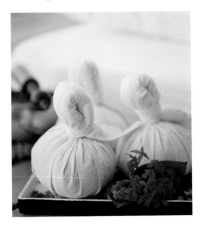
Healing herbal compress

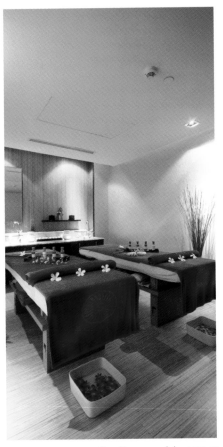
Spa Cenvaree deluxe room

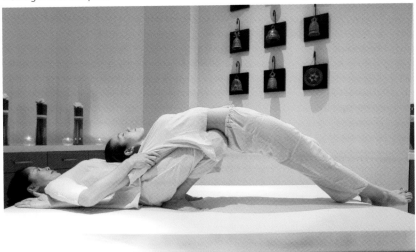
Royal Thai Massage treatment

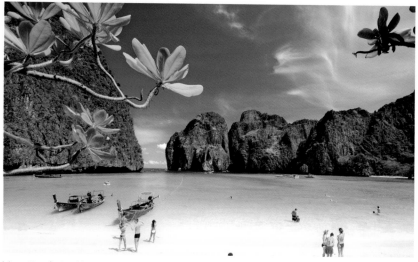

Maya Beach, Krabi

Cool ocean
breezes
surrounded by
white sandy
beaches.

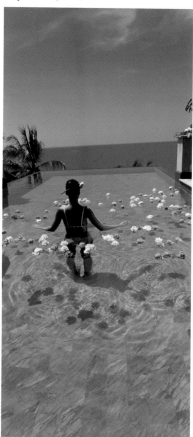

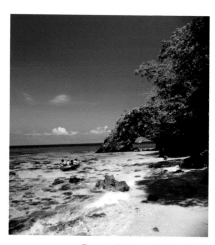

Rimless pool and deep blue sea

Tarutao National Park, Satun

Take Care Beauty Salon & Spa

J Avenue
Sukhumvit 55, 3rd Floor (Soi Thonglo)
Bangkok, THAILAND 10110
Tel: 66 2 712.6750

Take Care offers spa services with an emphasis on beauty. Separate facilities specialize in several different treatments:

✦ The hair section provides cut, color, perm, straightening, and extensions.

✦ In the nail treatment section, trained specialists provide manicure, pedicure, polishing, and nail extensions.

✦ The spa section provides spa treatment for face and body, including waxing.

✦ The massage section offers both body and foot massage.

✦ In the facial section, services include eyelash extensions, eyelash perm, eyebrow tinting, lip tinting, and make-up.

In the spa section, the aestheticians are specialists with as much as ten years' experience. Treatments use a variety of well-regarded spa product lines, including Decleor and Thalgo, in combination with natural and herbal therapies.

Type: Day

Signature Services

✦ Aroma Massage

✦ Skin Regenerating Herbal Scrub and Massage

✦ UMO Gold Facial (gold is said to stimulate collagen production)

Cost: An Aroma Massage starts at 1,000 baht (about US$30). The UMO Gold Facial costs 3,800 baht (about US$112) for 90 minutes.

TRIA Integrative Wellness

998 Rimkhlong Samsen Road
Bangkapi, Huai Khwang
Bangkok, THAILAND 10310
Tel: 66 2 660.2600
Fax: 66 2 660.2601
Email: info@triaintegrativewellness.com
Web: www.triaintegrativewellness.com

This spa has a distinctly medical bent: along with physicians, TRIA Integrative Wellness has a naturopath, chiropractor, nutritionist, and acupuncturist on staff, as well as specialists in Ayurvedic medicine, Japanese shiatsu, and moxibustion. Specialists consult with the client and prescribe everything from exercise regimens to colonic hydrotherapy.

TRIA staff members assert that wellness springs from the harmony of three essential health components: elemental, structural, and emotional states. Their teams take a holistic approach to health, optimizing services to meet individual needs. Services include fitness training, massage, various forms of hydrotherapy, and beautifying treatments. Package programs are available for movement and fitness, weight management, postnatal care, antiaging, holistic detoxification, mind and emotions, and rapid recovery. TRIA also offers cooking classes, meal packages, and tests for food allergies.

Type: Day

Signature Services

✦ Balancing Act: Integrative Medicine Consultation (one-hour diagnostic assessment)

✦ CryoStem Cell Medical Facial (bovine-origin stem cells to rejuvenate the skin)

✦ Go with the Flow: Manual Lymphatic Drainage (manual draining of stagnant body fluids with subtle maneuvers to activate lymph and interstitial fluid circulation)

Awards

✦ Best Day Spa, *SpaAsia* Crystal Awards, 2008

✦ Medi-Spa of the Year, *AsiaSpa* Awards, 2008

✦ Hot List Spas, *Condé Nast Traveller,* 2008

Cost: TRIA massages start at 2,800 baht (about US$82). The CryoStem Cell Medical Facial requires a prescription and costs 6,500 baht (about US$190).

OUTSIDE BANGKOK: HUA HIN

Hua Hin is located approximately 120 miles (about 200 kilometers) southwest of Bangkok. It's Thailand's oldest beach resort area, having attracted visitors since a railway line between Hua Hin and the capital first opened in the 1920s. Thai Royal Family members still customarily spend vacations there. We feature two spas in Hua Hin: Chiva-Som International Health Resort and Six Senses Spa at Evason.

Chiva-Som International Health Resort

734 Phetchakasem Road
Hua Hin
Prachuap Khiri Khan, THAILAND 77110
Tel: 66 32 53.6536
Fax: 66 32 51.1154
Email: sunisa.c@chivasom.com
Web: www.chivasom.com

Chiva-Som International Health Resort is situated on 7 beachfront acres (nearly 3 hectares) of lush tropical gardens, complete with views of the Gulf of Thailand. Chiva-Som offers fitness, spa, and holistic health services, combining ancient therapies of the East with modern Western techniques. Personalized programs drawn from more than 150 available treatments address weight management, stress reduction, skin rejuvenation, and aging. Fitness programs include tai chi, Pilates, personal training, and yoga. On staff are consulting doctors, naturopaths, fitness instructors, spa therapists, nutritionists, and alternative health practitioners.

Facilities include outdoor treatment spaces, a bathing pavilion, a beachfront swimming pool, multilevel steam rooms, plunge pools, hydro pools, a Watsu pool, an air-conditioned gym, and more. Spa cuisine uses organically grown fruits and vegetables from the Chiva-Som garden.

This is a residential spa, with customized retreats priced according to length of stay and residential preferences. All retreats include

✦ a health and wellness consultation on arrival

✦ three meals a day

✦ a daily massage

✦ participation in daily fitness and leisure activities

✦ complimentary use of steam room, sauna, and Jacuzzi

Type: Destination, with length of stay 3–28 days

Signature Services

✦ Chiva-Som's Skin-Smoothing Salt Scrub (fresh sea salts combined with oils of cinnamon and clove to assist circulation and soften skin)

✦ Oriental Foot Ritual (reflex point massage, exfoliation, footbath, and steamed herb-infused wrap)

✦ Skin Haven Facial (prepared from sugarcane, rain forest honey, aloe, and Thai herbs)

Awards

✦ Top Three Destination Spas, *Condé Nast Traveller* UK Readers Choice Awards, 1998–2008

✦ World's Best Destination Spa, *Travel+Leisure* Readers Choice Awards, 2006

✦ Spa Academy of the Year, *AsiaSpa* Awards, 2006

✦ Best Wellness Retreat and Best Complementary and Alternative Medicine Wellness Center, *SpaAsia* Crystal Awards, 2006

✦ Best Spa Academy, *SpaAsia* Crystal Awards, 2007

✦ Sixth Place, Top 15 Destination Spas, *Travel+Leisure* World's Best Awards, 2007

✦ Spa Cuisine of the Year, *AsiaSpa* Awards, 2008

✦ Top 10 Spas in Asia, SpaFinder.com, 2009

Cost: Prices of retreat packages range from an ocean-view single for three nights in the low season at US$1,860 to the Leelawadee Suite double for 28 nights in the high season at US$68,040.

Six Senses Spa

(At Evason Hua Hin)
9 Mu 5
Paknampran Beach, Pranburi
Prachuap Khiri Khan, THAILAND 77220
Tel: 66 32 63.2111
Fax: 66 32 63.2112
Email: reservations-huahin@sixsenses.com
Web: www.sixsenses.com

Evason Hua Hin is located in the quiet area of Pranburi, to the south of Hua Hin. This five-star resort boasts calming views of the Gulf of Thailand on 20 acres (about 8 hectares) of landscaped tropical gardens complete with lotus ponds. For ultimate relaxation, guests can stay in luxurious pool villas offering an outdoor bathtub sunken in a lily pond, a plush outdoor seating pavilion, and a private plunge pool. The facility's Six Senses Spa, adjacent to the beach, is noted for its innovative, nature-oriented design.

Focused on both pampering and healing, the spa offers a complete menu of therapeutic treatments and lifestyle programs, including wellness sessions featuring yoga and tai chi. Emphasizing eco-friendly practices and natural treatments, Six Senses is known as a leader in environmentally friendly spa development and operation.

Additional Locations in Thailand

Two in Phuket:

> Six Senses Destination Spa Phuket
> 32 Mu 5
> Paklok, Thalang
> Phuket, THAILAND 83110
> Tel: 66 76 37.1400
> Fax: 66 76 37.1401
> Email: reservations-naka@sixsenses.com

> Evason Phuket & Six Senses Spa
> 100 Wiset Road
> Mu 2
> Rawai, Mueang
> Phuket, THAILAND 83130
> Tel: 66 76 38.1010
> Fax: 66 76 38.1018
> Email: reservations-phuket@sixsenses.com

Type: Resort

Treatment Rooms: Outdoors, five rooms, each surrounded by lotus ponds; indoors, two couple rooms, four single rooms, two dry sauna rooms, two steam rooms

Signature Services

✦ Balancing Journey (body polish with clay wrap, Swedish massage, and facial)

✦ Energizing Journey (body toner, energizing massage, and foot acupressure)

✦ Sensory Journey (two therapists perform simultaneous facial and body massage)

Awards

✦ Fourth Place, Hotel Spas in Asia and Indian Subcontinent, *Condé Nast Traveller* UK Readers Choice Awards, 2006

✦ Silver Award, Most Popular Hotel/Resort in Southeast Asia, *Holidays for Couples* Readers Choice Awards, 2006

✦ Fifth Place, Favorite Overseas Hotel Spa in Asia, *Condé Nast Traveller* UK Readers Choice Awards, 2008

Cost: The Balancing Journey is priced at 6,600 baht (about US$194). The Sensory Journey costs 8,000 baht (about US$235).

OUTSIDE BANGKOK: KHAO YAI

Established in 1962 as Thailand's first national park, Khao Yai National Park encompasses a variety of landscapes in its mountains, waterfalls, evergreen forests, and grasslands. Hikers and nature lovers visit the area in hopes of spotting black bears, elephants, wild pigs, and the occasional tiger. Together with other parks in the Dong Phaya Yen Mountains, Khao Yai was declared a World Heritage Site by the United Nations Educational, Scientific, and Cultural Organization (UNESCO) in 2005. The park is about 98 miles (about 160 kilometers) from Bangkok, reachable by bus or train.

Maya Spa

(At Kirimaya Resort)
13 Mu 6
Thanarat Road
Mu 4, Pakchong
Nakhon Ratchasima, THAILAND 30130
Tel: 66 44 42.6000
Fax: 66 44 92.9888
Email: info@kirimaya.com
Web: www.kirimaya.com/resort

Open since 2004, Kirimaya Golf Resort and Spa is a high-end nature retreat nestled at the edge of Khao Yai National Park. Just two hours outside of Bangkok, this retreat is popular due to a cooler climate, diversity of wildlife, and breathtaking vistas. Kirimaya's 60 rooms and suites are elegantly designed, incorporating natural materials and emphasizing the park's exceptional beauty. Recently referred to as "glamping," a stay in the tented villas is a special treat combining easy style with upscale amenities.

"The Kirimaya experience" includes the Maya Spa, food service, and a Jack Nicklaus–designed 18-hole championship golf course. The wellness spa offers facial and body treatments, therapeutic baths, wellness packages, and in-room massage. Selected treatments incorporate grapes from the nearby vineyard and the resort's organic gardens.

Type: Resort

Treatment Rooms: Four cooled rooms, one cooled Thai massage room

Signature Services

✦ Detox Treatment (massage with grape seed oil and soak in Thai herbal bath salts)

✦ Jet Lag Reliever (foot bath and scrub, aromatherapy massage, and face/scalp/foot massage)

✦ Khao Yai Therapy (grape therapy body scrub, wine wrap, wine and grape juice bath, Kirimaya massage, and organic grape facial)

Cost: The two-hour Jet Lag Reliever is priced at 3,200 baht (about US$94). A 90-minute Kirimaya massage costs 2,900 baht (about US$85).

OUTSIDE BANGKOK: NAKHON PATHOM

Nakhon Pathom is a small province located in the alluvial plain of central Thailand, about 36 miles (60 kilometers) west of Bangkok. Its main provincial city bears the same name and is one of the oldest in Thailand, with structures in the area dating back to 200 BC. Visitors come to see the Phra Pathom Chedi, erected by Theravada Buddhists in the sixth century; it is the tallest Buddhist monument in the world and the oldest in Thailand. We feature one spa in Nakhon Pathom.

Arusaya Spa

Km 32 Phetchakasem Road
Sampran
Nakhon Pathom, THAILAND 73110
Tel: 66 34 32.5478
Fax: 66 34 32.2775
Email: hotel@rosegardenriverside.com
Web: www.rosegardenriverside.com

Arusaya Spa is located at the Rose Garden Riverside, a 70-acre (28-hectare) botanical park about 60 miles (100 kilometers) from Bangkok. The site features jasmine, orchids, roses, banana plants, rare native plant species, and therapeutic herbs. Lucky visitors sometimes spot elephants, buffalo, and flamingos. The site also includes six restored century-old teak houses, which are set on stilts next to expertly cultivated gardens and a man-made lake. Accommodations are available in the Rose Garden Riverside Hotel or in the antique houses.

Arusaya is a boutique Thai spa. Set in a serene herb garden and located in a century-old Thai house, treatments feature fresh-picked herbal compresses from the garden and custom-selected essential oils. Certified therapists and trained Thai traditional medicine experts provide massage and facial treatments. Lessons in Thai herbal medicine are available.

Type: Hotel/resort

Treatment Rooms: Seven air-conditioned rooms (en-suite with bathrooms), three steam rooms

Signature Services

✦ Arusaya Royal Herbal Treatment

✦ Arusaya Sport Massage

✦ Facial Harmonization Facial

✦ Rose Garden Revival Massage

Cost: The Facial Harmonization Facial costs 1,400 baht (about US$41), as does the 80-minute Rose Garden Revival Massage.

IN PHUKET

Phuket (pronounced pooh-GET) is the largest and best known of Thailand's islands, and a popular destination for vacationers. Its beaches and forests attract sightseers from all over the world. It's a paradise for water sports enthusiasts, and its resorts are among the most luxurious anywhere. Phuket has developed and overdeveloped its tourist areas—especially in Patong—so if you're looking for peace and quiet, choose carefully. We feature three spas in Phuket that may help you wind down.

Banyan Tree Spa Phuket

33 Mu 4
Srisunthorn Road
Cherngtalay, Thalang
Phuket, THAILAND 83110
Tel: 66 76 32.4374
Fax: 66 76 27.1463
Email: spa-phuket@banyantree.com
Web: www.banyantreespa.com

Banyan Tree Spa Phuket opened in 1994 as Asia's first luxury spa resort, pioneering the tropical garden spa concept. Its packages integrate Eastern therapies and a holistic focus on spiritual, mental, and physical harmony. Banyan Tree emphasizes a "low-tech, high-touch" approach and the use of natural herbs and spices. The spa has its own academy, where its therapists are trained to administer massages, body scrubs and conditioning treatments, facials and other beauty regiments, and Ayurvedic remedies. Staff members also provide instruction in yoga and Pilates. Resort facilities include a golf club, outdoor pool, tennis courts, and art gallery. Banyan Tree operates other spa retreats in Bahrain, China, Indonesia, Japan, the Maldives, and the Seychelles.

Additional Locations in Thailand

One in Bangkok:

> Banyan Tree Spa Bangkok
> Thai Wah Tower II, 21st Floor
> Sathon Road
> Bangkok, THAILAND 10120
> Tel: 66 2 679.1052
> Fax: 66 2 679.1053
> Email: spa-bangkok@banyantree.com
> Web: www.banyantreespa.com

Type: Destination/resort

Treatment Rooms: Twenty-five rooms

Signature Services

✦ Master Therapist Experience (90-minute massage by an expert therapist)

✦ Rainmist Experience (steam bath, shower, and massage)

✦ Royal Banyan Herbal Pouch Massage (massage with an herbal pouch dipped in warm sesame oil)

Awards

✦ World's Best Spa Resort, *Condé Nast Traveler* Readers Choice Awards, 1999

✦ World's Top Ten Hotel Spas, *Travel+Leisure,* 2000

Cost: The Master Therapist Experience is priced at 5,200 baht (about US$152). The Royal Banyan Herbal Pouch Massage costs 8,500 baht (about US$249).

Royal Spa

(At Absolute Sea Pearl Resort)
421 Thaweewong Road
Patong Beach
Phuket, THAILAND 83150
Tel: 66 76 34.1901
Fax: 66 76 34.1122
Email: info@theroyalspa.com; info@absoluteseapearl.com
Web: www.theroyalspa.com; www.absoluteseapearl.com

Absolute Sea Pearl, one of the best-known hotels in Phuket, is only a few steps off Patong Beach. It lies within easy walking distance of shopping, entertainment, and Phuket's raucous nightlife. The Royal Spa's facilities include an herbal steam bath, rain shower, and luxury bath. The Royal Spa chain operates its own training academy in medical and alternative therapies; its program is approved by the Ministry of Education and accredited by the International Center of Chiang Mai University. Royal Spa also operates in 14 other Thai hotels.

Type: Resort/hotel

Signature Services

✦ Royal Ayurvedic Massage (full-body and scalp massage with medicated oils)

✦ Royal Experience Massage (full-body massage with specially created massage oil)

✦ Royal Signature Package (four-hour bath, body wrap, facial, and massage)

✦ Royal Stone Therapy (hot stone massage)

Treatment Rooms: Three rooms

Cost: The Royal Experience Massage costs 1,850 baht (about US$54). The Royal Signature Package is priced at 5,600 baht (about US$164).

Sukko Cultural Spa & Wellness

510 Mu 3
Wichit, Mueang
Phuket, THAILAND 83000
Tel: 66 76 26.3222
Fax: 66 76 26.4533
Email: sukko@sukkospa.com
Web: www.sukkospa.com

Sukko Cultural Spa & Wellness calls itself "the world's first cultural spa" for a reason. Its "cultural wellness" programs involve visitors in a range of learning activities that include Thai cooking classes, Ashtanga yoga, aqua exercise, and Thai arts and crafts, such as fruit and vegetable carving, hair braiding, jasmine garland-making, and much more. To get the blood flowing and the brain working, there's the martial art of Muai Thai Chaiya and the traditional Thai exercise of Rue Sri Datton, which combines stretching and applying pressure to energy points with breathing techniques and meditation. All the modern conveniences are on offer, too. The Suk Sanan Club House is equipped with state-of-the-art exercise equipment and complete with plasma TV and wireless Internet. Members are free to use the herbal steam rooms, saunas, Jacuzzi, ozone-treated pool, and activity room.

The spa offers 40 individualized spa packages requiring two to four hours. À la carte treatments include scrubs, body wraps, aromatherapy baths, heat treatments, facials, manicures, salon services, and massages. Herbal recipes and procedures handed down through generations ensure that Sukko products are free of petrochemicals, synthetic perfumes, or colors.

Additional Locations in Thailand

Sukko Spas operate at 12 other hotels in Thailand, including this one in Phuket:

> Sukko Spa
> (At Khaolak Seaview Resort)
> 181 Mu 7
> Nangthong Beach, Phetchakasem Road
> Kukkak, Khaolak
> Takuapa, Phang Nga, THAILAND 82190
> Tel: 66 76 42.9800
> Fax: 66 76 42.9819

Type: Day

Signature Services

✦ Energy Rebalance (Thai coffee body scrub, traditional Thai massage, and foot massage)

✦ Princess-to-Be (four-hour steam/Jacuzzi, rice body scrub, aromatherapy massage, facial, and manicure/pedicure with nail art)

✦ Style of Silk (steam/Jacuzzi, herbal salt body scrub, aromatherapy massage, and facial)

Awards (for Sukko Spas)

✦ Award of Excellence, Day Spa, Thailand Tourism Awards, 2008

✦ Outstanding Performance in Health Tourism, Day Spa, Thailand Tourism Awards, 2008–2009

✦ Awards for Excellence, Spa of the Year, and Best Signature Day Spa in Southeast Asia, Hospitality Asia Platinum Awards, 2008–2010

Cost: An à la carte Ayurvedic massage costs 2,800 baht (about US$82). The Princess-to-Be package costs 5,300 baht (about US$155).

Traveling in Thailand

International travel can be a life-changing experience, and medical travelers can bring back more from their trip than improved health—they can return with an appreciation for a landscape, a culture, and a way of life very different from their own. In Thailand, international patients and their companions can take advantage of the opportunity to sample the sights, sounds, and flavors of urban Bangkok, the tropical beaches of Phuket, or the forests and wildlife of Khao Yai National Park.

Part Four provides important details to help you plan your medical journey to Thailand—along with some ideas for enjoying the country's unique sights and experiences while you're there.

Thailand in Brief

Thailand is situated in the heart of the Southeast Asian mainland, bordering the Lao People's Democratic Republic (Lao PDR) and the Union of Myanmar (Burma) to the north; the Kingdom of Cambodia and Lao PDR to the east; the Union of Myanmar and the Andaman Sea to the west; and Malaysia and the Gulf of Thailand to the south. Its capital is Bangkok. Thailand's other major cities are Chiang Mai (north); Songkhla (south); Ayutthaya and Chonburi (central); and Nakhon Ratchasima and Khon Kaen (northeastern).

Opinions differ as to the origins of the Thai people. Three decades ago, experts were more or less certain that the Thais originated in northwestern Sichuan in China about 4,500 years ago and later migrated south to their present homeland. However, the discovery of some remarkable prehistoric artifacts in the village of Ban Chiang in the northeastern province of Udon

Thani has called that theory into question. These artifacts provide evidence of bronze metallurgy going back 3,500 years, as well as other indications of a far more sophisticated culture than was previously suspected by archaeologists. It now appears that the Thais might have originated in Thailand and later scattered to various parts of Asia, including some parts of China.

Thailand was called Siam until 1939 and again between 1945 and 1949. On May 11, 1949, an official proclamation changed the name of the country to Prathet Thai, or Thailand, by which it has since been known. The word *thai* means "free"; therefore, Thailand means "the Land of the Free." Unofficially, it's known as "the Land of Smiles" because of the renowned hospitality of the Thai people.

Bangkok, "the City of Angels," became the capital in 1782, with the founding of the Chakri Dynasty that still occupies the Thai throne. Many of the city's landmarks date from this period, among them the magnificent Grand Palace and its adjacent temples of Wat Phra Kaeo, Wat Arun, and Wat Pho. Rivers and canals were the traditional means of transport in Bangkok, and no roads were built until the 1860s—it was the network of rivers and canals that led early European visitors to describe the city as "the Venice of the East." Today it's a sprawling metropolis of high-rise buildings, shopping centers, boutique residences, and world-class luxury hotels.

Whether you allot a day, a week, or a month for seeing the sights of Thailand, you'll never run out of things to do. In this section, we feature only attractions in Bangkok and Phuket, because most medical travelers stay there. If you have a chance to venture farther, check with the international patient center at your hospital, the service desk at your hotel, or any good travel guidebook for ideas galore. Thailand is truly the Land of Smiles, a country of ancient culture, historic temples and palaces, stunning scenery, and charming hospitality. Take time to enjoy a little of it all.

Ten Things to Do
While in Thailand

1. Sample the City of Gourmet Delights

✦ Yaowarat: Bangkok's Chinatown boasts some of the best Chinese restaurants in the city, along with many of the best and cheapest food stalls, especially at night.

✦ Sukhumvit: Sukhumvit Soi 55 offers everything from sidewalk noodle stalls to trendy air-conditioned restaurants serving international cuisine.

✦ Silom: This is the busiest area of Bangkok, with cafés, bistros, and food stalls offering French, Korean, Japanese, Italian, Swiss, Californian, Irish, and Thai cuisines.

✦ Riverside: Great places to dine dot the riverbank from the Rama IX Bridge to Phra Nang Klao Bridge in Nonthaburi— or try a dinner cruise.

✦ Lang Suan: This is a boulevard of smart new restaurants in an up-market residential and commercial area.

✦ Bang Lamphu-Khao San: The bars and restaurants of the Bang Lamphu area and Khao San Road are favorites among young, budget-conscious travelers.

✦ Phahurat: Known as Bangkok's Little India, Phahurat is home to many authentic Indian and Pakistani restaurants.

2. Shop 'til you drop

Bangkok offers a wealth of modern, state-of-the-art shopping malls as well as department stores, plazas, and exclusive outlets. Shoppers will find top fashion stores with global brand names, specialty stores for high-tech equipment, and boutiques offering every kind of luxury lifestyle product, plus bookshops, gourmet food outlets, and special attractions. Most shopping complexes are easily accessible via the Bangkok Transit System (BTS) Sky Train network.

Every year from the beginning of June until the end of August, the TAT-organized Amazing Thailand Grand Sale campaign provides visitors opportunities to shop at special promotional prices. Or you can try bargain hunting at Chatuchak Weekend Market, where 9,000 booths sell an infinite variety of goods every Saturday and Sunday—it's nearly impossible to leave without buying something.

Travel Fun in Thailand

For more ideas on things to see and do in Thailand, visit the official Web site of the Tourism Authority of Thailand (TAT) at www.tourismthailand.org.

3. Ride a river taxi or take a canal tour

Old Bangkok was a city of waterways, the greatest being the Chao Phraya River, "the River of Kings." Today it still supports a colorful, commercial river life with long trains of slow-moving traditional barges, fast long-tail boats, river taxis, and the regular cross-river ferries to and from riverside hotels. Taking a cruise along this legendary river and some canals on the Thonburi side is a pleasant way to explore the city's origins and way of life.

4. Learn a little history

For an unusual exploration of the ethnology, anthropology, and history of Thailand's people, society, and relationships within Southeast Asia, visit the Museum Siam Discovery Museum, where modern media displays will entice you into exhibit rooms on subjects ranging from village life to Bangkok, from war to Buddhism, and from ancient maps to the nation's future. At the National Museum, exhibits reveal how people lived during Thailand's various historical periods, and the Bangkok Folk Museum features a recreation of a World War II–era family home in Bangkok.

5. Admire some art and architecture

Phra Thinang Chakri Maha Prasat, the royal residence built in 1877 by King Rama V, is Thailand's most widely recognized architectural landmark. The Arts of the Kingdom Museum at the Ananda Samakhom Throne Hall displays traditional arts from each region of the country. The Vimanmek Mansion is an outstanding example of nineteenth-century architecture and craftsmanship. Enormous replicas of Thailand's most famous buildings, monuments, and temples are featured at the 280-acre (113-hectare) Ancient City, the largest outdoor museum in the world.

6. Visit a religious site

The Grand Palace, also known as Wat Phra Kaeo or "the Temple of the Emerald Buddha," is a "must-visit" site in Bangkok. Visitors also flock to Wat Arun, "the Temple of Dawn," and Wat Benchamabophit, "the Marble Temple." The famed Wat Pho, "the Temple of the Reclining Buddha," is a center for meditation and traditional Thai massage training.

7. Appreciate the performing arts

Siam Niramit is a one-of-a-kind cultural theme complex, offering performances of Thailand's arts and cultural heritage in a 2,000-seat theater. Visitors to the Joe Louis Puppet Theater will see the last of the kingdom's traditional Thai small puppets troupes. One of the most refined of the performing arts is the Khon Masked Dance at Sala Chalermkrung Theater; originally limited to the royal court, its performances feature lavish costumes, elaborate masks and headgear, and skillfully crafted stage accessories.

8. Marvel at some animal life

Siam Ocean World is the largest aquarium in Southeast Asia, spanning more than 107,600 square feet (about 10,000 square meters) full of aquatic life and offering daily feeding shows. At Safari World, visitors can get close to wild animals roaming free in a 170-acre (69-hectare) park.

9. View a sporting event

Boxing enthusiasts may wish to take in a bout of Muai Thai (Thai boxing), while soccer fans may want to get tickets for the Thailand King's Cup International Football Tournament, held each December. International Swan Boat Races run on the Chao Phraya River in September, the same month that competitors in the Vertical Marathon prove their mettle by running up 61 flights of stairs. Bangkok also hosts a wide variety of tennis tournaments, along with numerous cycling, running, kayaking, and swimming competitions.

10. Enjoy the beaches, parks, and golf courses of Phuket

Hat Patong is the most developed—some might say over-developed—most vibrant, and most visited beach of Phuket. Located approximately 9 miles (15 kilometers) from Phuket City, the beach offers a wide range of accommodations, shopping pavilions, leisure activities, and nighttime entertainment. With nearly 2 miles (3 kilometers) of white sand, the beach is perfect for swimming, sunbathing, jet skiing, windsurfing, snorkeling, sailing, and parasailing, but Patong is probably best known for its nightlife, noise, and alternative lifestyles. Most medical travelers opt instead for an inexpensive 30-minute taxi ride to any of the numerous quieter beaches along Phuket's coastline. Sirinat National Park, about 19 miles (30 kilometers) from the city, features mangrove forests and an 8-mile (13-kilometer) beach. Golfers will find plenty of attractive courses on Phuket, too.

Thai Cuisine

Exotic flavors abound in Thailand, and each region offers its own culinary specialties. From tantalizing packages at roadside stalls to platters at fine restaurants, visitors can experience the country's many different cooking styles and distinctive ingredients. Look for . . .

. . . zesty dips made from chilies, garlic, onion, shrimp paste, sour tamarind, and more.

. . . spicy salads dressed with fish sauce, lime juice, and sugar, and garnished with fresh mint, lemongrass, Kaffir lime leaves, or coriander.

. . . smooth curries blending chili, garlic, shallot, galangal, coriander root, and *krachai* (a root indigenous to Thailand). In Thai curries, the curry paste is cooked in coconut cream before the meat or vegetables are added, so they tend to be milder than Indian curries.

. . . desserts often made from eggs and coconut milk and complemented with Thai fruits, such as banana, mango, lychee, rambutan, mangosteen, and durian. The famous dish of mango and sticky rice is not to be missed!

On restaurant menus, look for these "top ten" specialties:

- *Tom yam kung* (spicy shrimp soup)
- *Kaeng khieo wan kai* (chicken green curry)
- *Phat Thai* (Thai fried noodles)
- *Phat kaphrao* (meat fried with sweet basil)
- *Kaeng phet pet yang* (roast duck curry)
- *Tom kha kai* (chicken in coconut soup)
- *Yam nua* (spicy beef salad)
- *Mu* or *kai sa-te* (roast pork or chicken coated with turmeric)
- *Kai phat met mamuang himmaphan* (chicken fried with cashew nuts)
- *Phanaeng* (meat in coconut cream)

The Medical Traveler's Essentials

This section provides a handy rundown of practical information on transportation, currency, communications, and other "nuts and bolts" of travel to Thailand.

Geography

Thailand, the hub of Southeast Asia, is bordered by Malaysia, Myanmar, Lao PDR, and Cambodia, thus making it the natural gateway to the Greater Mekong subregion of Asia. Each of Thailand's four distinct regions—Central, South, North, and Northeast—has its own unique natural and cultural attributes.

Climate

Most of Thailand enjoys a relatively comfortable tropical climate in three distinct seasons:

- Summer is March–May, with hot, dry weather and temperatures averaging 82–91°F (28–33°C).
- The southwest monsoon season is mid-May to September, wet but with plenty of sunshine and a temperature range of 80–86°F (27–30°C).
- Temperatures cool a bit in October, and the northeast monsoon season is November–February, mild and wet but still very sunny with temperatures 75–80°F (24–27°C).

Medical travelers to Thailand generally avoid the period of March–June, when the Thai heat may not be conducive to the most comfortable recovery.

Time Zone

Thailand is seven hours ahead of Greenwich Mean Time (GMT+7).

Population and Ethnicity

The diversity of Thailand's 65.5 million people reflects the nation's history. While three-quarters are Thai, 14 percent are of Chinese heritage, and 11 percent are of Malay, Laotian, Indian, or Burmese extraction.

Languages

Spoken Thai is a tonal language of the Ka-Tai linguistic group, with written Thai having its roots in Pali and Sanskrit. Even so, visitors to Thailand won't have communication problems. English is widely understood—especially in Bangkok, where it is a major commercial language—and Thai-English street signs are used nationwide. Chinese, French, German, Japanese, and Spanish are also spoken in most hotels, shops, and restaurants in major tourist destinations.

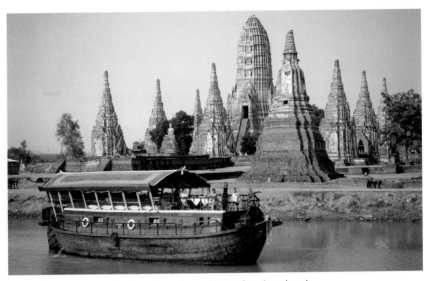

The Mekhala, a former rice barge transformed into a boutique hotel

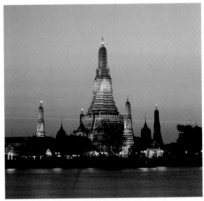

Wat Arun, Temple of Dawn

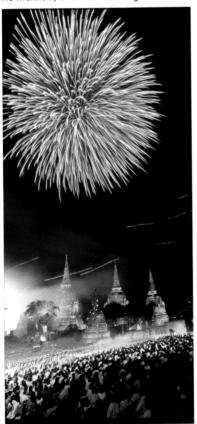

One of Thailand's many World Heritage sites

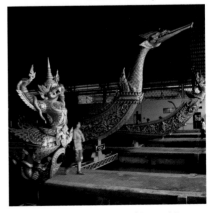

Royal Barge Museum

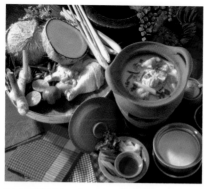

Kha gai (chicken in coconut soup)

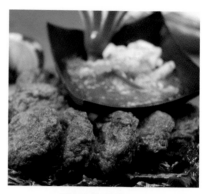

Thot mun (fish or prawn cakes)

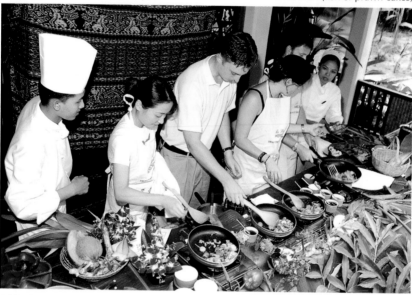

Sukhothai cooking class

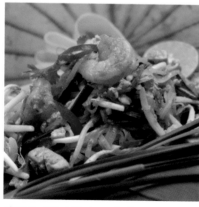

Phat Thai (Thai fried noodles)

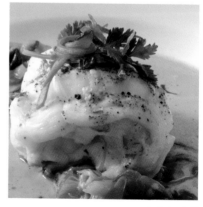

Lobster tail

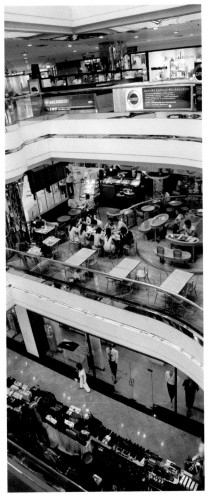

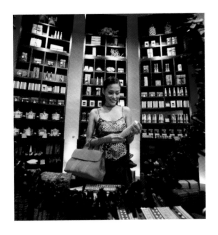

Bangkok offers
an array of
shopping from
quaint markets
to upscale
malls and
plazas.

Dozens of modern malls welcome shoppers

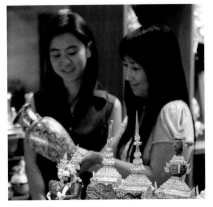

Local crafts and artifacts

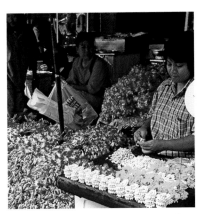

One of Thailand's famous flower markets

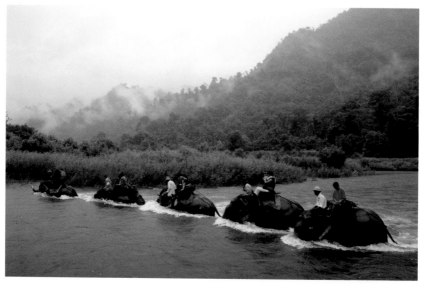
Elephant trekking, Northern Thailand

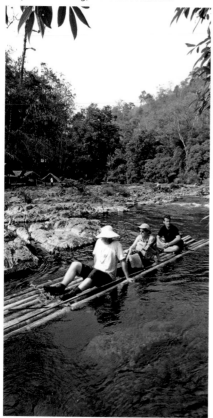

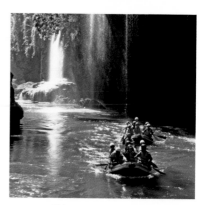
Thi Lo Re Waterfall, Tak province

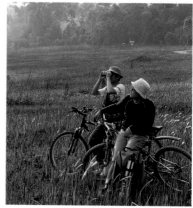

Rafting, Northern Thailand

Birdwatching in a Thai national park

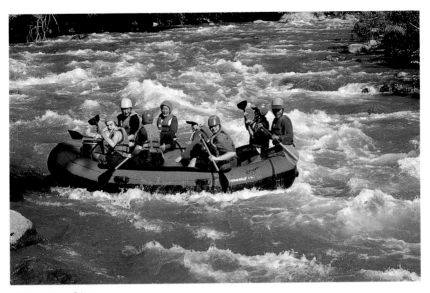
Whitewater rafting

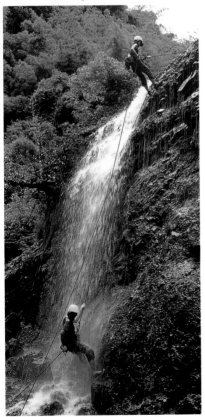

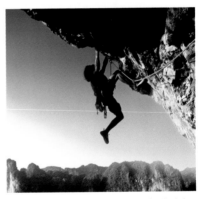
Scaling the heights

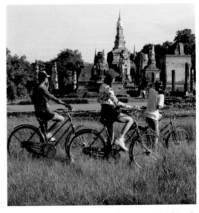

Rock climbing

Biking in Sukhothai Historical Park

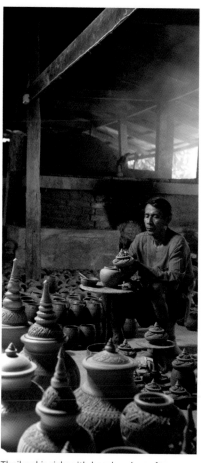

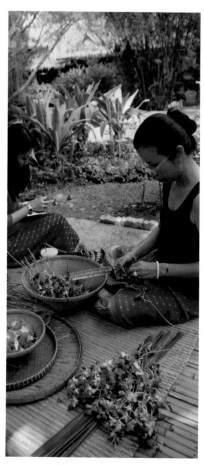

Thailand is rich with handmade crafts

Preparing orchids for the market

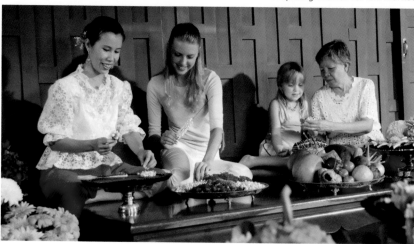

Living the Thai culture

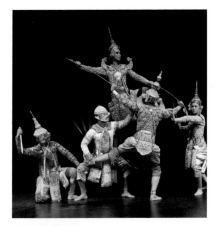

Khon Masked Dance

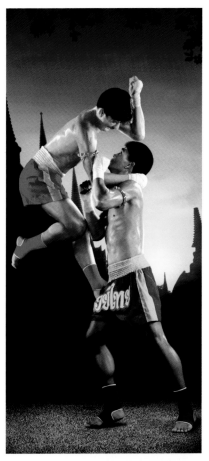

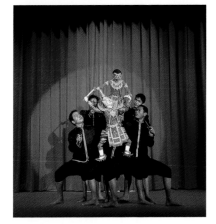

Joe Louis Puppet Theater

Muai Thai, "the art of eight limbs"

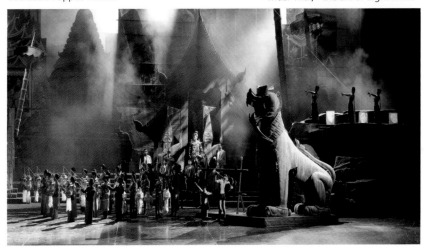

Siam Niramit

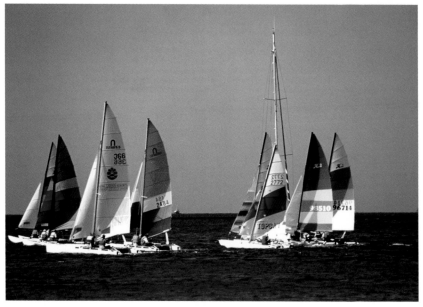

Sailing on the Gulf of Thailand

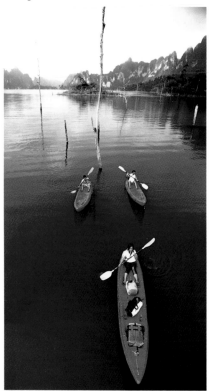

Thailand offers
a variety
of coastal
recreational
activities.

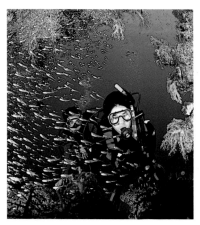

Kayaking off the southern coast

Diving in a Thai marine park

Dress Code

Light, cool, loose cotton clothing is the best for Thailand's tropical climate. Sweaters are recommended when visiting the northern mountainous region and national parks during the cool season. Shorts (except knee-length walking shorts), sleeveless shirts, tank tops, and other beach-style attire are considered inappropriate dress when not actually at the beach or a resort area. When visiting Buddhist temples, long pants are required. Always remember to remove your shoes before entering a temple or a Thai person's home or room.

Electricity

The electric current throughout Thailand is 220-volt AC (50 cycles), but many different types of plugs and sockets are in use. Travelers bringing shavers, hair dryers, tape recorders, and other electrical appliances should carry a plug adapter kit. Large hotels usually have 110-volt transformers available for guests.

Passport and Visa

All visitors to Thailand are required to possess a passport valid for at least six months after the date of arrival. Citizens of 41 countries and Hong Kong do not need a visa when entering Thailand for stays of less than 30 days. Citizens of 21 other countries can apply for a visa upon arrival at the immigration hall of any international airport in Thailand and at border checkpoints. Visitors from a number of other countries, however, need to obtain a visa from their nearest Thai embassy or consulate prior to their arrival in Thailand. For more information, see www.mfa.go.th.

Immunizations

Thai authorities require no inoculations, except for travelers arriving from or passing through a designated contaminated area. The US Centers for Disease Control and Prevention (CDC) recommend that all international travelers stay up-to-date with routine immunizations, which include influenza, chickenpox (or varicella), polio, measles/mumps/rubella (MMR), and diphtheria/pertussis/tetanus (DPT). Although childhood diseases, such as measles, rarely occur in the US today, they are not uncommon in many parts of the world, so an unvaccinated traveler is at risk for infection.

The CDC also recommends that all travelers who might be exposed to blood or other body fluids through medical treatment be immunized against hepatitis B. Immunization against hepatitis A and boosters for typhoid and polio are recommended as well. Travelers to Thailand's major cities do not need to take medicines to prevent malaria; there is, however, some risk of malaria in the rural areas that border Cambodia, Lao PDR, and Myanmar. For more information, check the CDC's Web site, wwwn.cdc.gov/travel/destinations/list.aspx.

Customs Regulations

Foreign visitors to Thailand may bring personal effects and other goods that are not prohibited by customs regulations. Visitors departing from Thailand are also allowed to take out merchandise bought from duty-free shops, including precious stones, gold, and platinum ornaments.

Personal items: Customs regulations allow visitors to bring a still camera, a video camera, 200 cigarettes or 250 grams of tobacco, and 1 liter of wine or spirits. Narcotics and pornography are strictly prohibited.

Professional items: The import of stationery items for use during conventions is not subject to import duties, nor is professional presentation equipment.

Currency Import/Export Regulations

- Tourists may freely bring foreign banknotes or other types of foreign exchange into Thailand.
- Upon leaving Thailand, tourists may take foreign currency with them, unless the amount exceeds either the equivalent of US$10,000 or the amount declared in writing to customs upon arrival.
- Foreign currency brought into or taken out of Thailand that exceeds the value of US$10,000 must be declared at the customs office. Failure to do so may lead to arrest, confiscation of funds, and/or prosecution.
- Travelers can take a maximum of 50,000 baht (about US$1,468) per person out of the country without authorization.
- Thai currency up to 500,000 baht (about US$14,674) can be taken to neighboring countries (Myanmar, Lao PDR, Cambodia, and Vietnam) without authorization.
- Nonresidents are allowed to open foreign currency accounts with any commercial bank in Thailand. No restrictions are imposed on these accounts, as long as funds originate from abroad.
- Foreign visitors may convert Thai baht into foreign currency for the purpose of outbound travel by presenting a currency exchange receipt, valid airline ticket, and passport at any major bank.

Airport Tax

Departing international travelers must pay a 700-baht tax (about US$21) levied by the national airport operator, Airports of Thailand. The cost may be included in a prepaid airline ticket, or it may be collected at a desk at the airport.

VAT Refund

Visitors entering on a tourist visa and departing through any of Thailand's international airports are entitled to a refund of the 7 percent value-added tax (VAT) on goods (except gemstones and items prohibited for export) purchased at registered retail outlets. Obtaining the refund involves a bit of planning. At the time of purchase, the buyer must present a passport, and the seller must complete a form and attach a receipt. Upon departure, the traveler must present the goods, the form, and the receipt to customs officers at the airport.

Currency

The Thai unit of currency, the baht, is not fixed to any other currency; it fluctuates with world market rates. It is based on the decimal system, with 1 baht divided into 100 satang. Coins are 25 and 50 satang and 1, 2, 5, and 10 baht. Paper notes are in 20-, 50-, 100-, 500-, and 1,000-baht denominations.

Traveler's Checks, Money Changing, and Credit Cards

Traveler's checks are generally accepted as payment at all hotels. Traveler's checks and currency notes in all major currencies may be exchanged at commercial banks, most hotels, and foreign exchange counters. Thai and foreign banks provide a standard service nationwide. US-dollar traveler's checks can also be cashed at provincial banks and authorized money changers; the best rates are in Bangkok.

Many first-class hotels provide 24-hour money exchange services, but only for a limited group of major currencies, such as the US dollar, euro, pound sterling, German mark, and Swiss franc. Hotel exchange rates are usually lower than those offered by banks and authorized money changers.

Major credit cards are widely accepted.

Banks and ATMs

Office hours for banks are generally 0830 to 1530 hours Monday through Friday, except on bank holidays and public holidays. Bank branches located in some major shopping malls are now open for most transactions until 2000 hours and on Saturday and Sunday as well. Major banks, such as Bangkok Bank,

Bank of Ayudhya, Kasikorn, Krung Thai, and Siam Commercial, have 24-hour ATM machines that accept all major debit and credit cards.

Postal Services

Major hotels provide basic postal services on their premises. Post offices nationwide are open Monday through Friday from 0800 to 1700 hours, and on Saturday from 0800 hours to midday. For more information, go to www .thailandpost.com.

Business Hours for Stores and Offices

Many stores are open seven days a week from 1000 to 2200 hours. Most private offices in Bangkok operate on a five-day week from 0800 to 1700 hours. Generally, government offices are open Monday through Friday from 0830 to 1630 hours (with a lunch break from noon to 1300 hours), except on public holidays.

Internet

Thailand offers Internet services in most leading hotels and in many cyber-cafés located throughout the country. If you need wireless Internet access, ask about its availability before making a hotel reservation.

Telecommunications

International telephone calls can be made easily from nearly every hotel in Thailand, via direct dialing for more than 80 countries. Special booths at post offices offer overseas calling services, and phone cards can be purchased in Bangkok and other tourist areas for use in international phone booths.

The international country code for Thailand is 66; domestic calls do not use the country code. All calls to landline phone numbers in Thailand use city codes. Domestic calls include an initial 0 in the city code—examples are 02 for Bangkok, 053 for Chiang Mai, and 076 for Phuket—whereas calls from outside the country do not (see instructions below).

International phone calls. When making an international call to a land-line in Thailand, dial the appropriate international access code, followed by the country code 66, then the city code *without* an initial 0, and then the phone number.

When making an international call from Thailand, dial the international access code 001, followed by the appropriate country code, then the area code, and then the phone number. Exceptions are calls from Thailand to Lao PDR or

Malaysia, which use a special code that's charged at a semidomestic rate: dial 007 + 856 + area code + phone number.

Domestic phone calls. When making either a local or a long-distance call within Thailand, dial the city code *with* an initial 0, followed by the phone number.

Mobile phones. Mobile phone numbers begin with the code 081, 083, 084, 085, 086, 087, 088, or 089, followed by the number. Subscriber Identity Module (SIM) cards for use with mobile phones are available to both Thais and foreign customers. A SIM card can be used with a digital GSM phone within the 900-megahertz range or a digital PCN phone within the 1,800-megahertz range.

Useful Telephone Numbers
- Local Directory Assistance: 1133 (Bangkok), 183 (upcountry)
- Overseas Directory Assistance: 100
- Police, Ambulance, Fire: 191
- Highway Patrol: 1193
- Crime Suppression: 195, 2 513.3844
- Tourist Police: 1155 (English, French, and German spoken)
- Tourism Authority of Thailand (TAT) Call Center: 1672
- Immigration Bureau: 2 287.3101

Tipping
Tipping is not a standard practice in Thailand, although it is becoming more so. Larger hotels and restaurants add a 10 percent service charge to the bill. Taxi drivers do not expect a tip, but the gesture is always appreciated. A tip of 20–50 baht is acceptable for porters. Tips should be given in baht, not foreign currency.

Smoking
Thailand has a national ban on smoking in public areas, including pubs, restaurants, discos, and marketplaces, both open air and air-conditioned. Violators can be fined as much as 2,000 baht (US$65). As a medical traveler, of course, you are strongly advised to stop smoking—but if you must smoke, look for the designated areas set aside for smokers.

Drinking Water
The tap water is clean but not recommended for drinking. Bottled water is best.

Transportation

Bangkok is Thailand's major gateway. International or domestic travel on public holidays and weekends, particularly to popular destinations, should be booked well in advance for all modes of transport. This is especially true during the Songkran Festival celebrating the Thai traditional New Year, April 13–15.

Air. Most visitors arrive at the new Suvarnabhumi International Airport, roughly 15 miles (about 25 kilometers) east of Bangkok. Flights arrive daily from Europe, Asia, North America, and Australia. Additional international flights— mainly from Singapore, Malaysia, and Hong Kong—land at the airports of Phuket and Hat Yai in the South and Chiang Mai in the North.

Flying within Thailand is inexpensive and convenient. The number of domestic airports has grown, all with connecting flights to Bangkok and at least one other destination. The quickest means of transport in Thailand is the domestic network operated by Thai Airways, which flies out of Bangkok to Chiang Mai, Chiang Rai, Hat Yai, Khon Kaen, Krabi, Nakhon Si Thammarat, Trang, Phitsanulok, Phuket, Surat Thani, Ubon Ratchathani, and Udon Thani.

Several independent and budget carriers, including Bangkok Airways, Air Asia, Nok Air, PB Air, and SGA Airlines, also have regular flights to locations within Thailand and overseas. Some airlines offer a range of tour packages for travelers. Reservations may be secured through airline offices, hotels, or travel agencies. Further details may be obtained on the airlines' call centers and Web sites.

Rail. Thailand is served by an extensive rail network using Bangkok as its hub. State Railway of Thailand (SRT) operates four train lines: Northern, Northeastern, Eastern, and Southern. Its train classifications are Special Express (the fastest), Express, Rapid, and Ordinary. Different classes of seating and amenities are available, so check ahead of time to ensure the comfort and convenience you desire. The SRT Web site is www.railway.co.th.

Regular SRT train service links Bangkok with Singapore via Kuala Lumpur and Butterworth in Malaysia. Trains depart daily and connect with many major southern Thai towns en route. The luxury Eastern & Oriental Express service runs from Chiang Mai to Bangkok, then southward across the border to Malaysia, and on to Singapore.

For 15 baht (about 45 US cents), the Bangkok Mass Transit Authority (BMTA, www.transport.co.th) provides shuttle bus service linking Suvarnabhumi International Airport with Hua Takhe Railway Station on SRT's Eastern Line. SRT provides suburban commuter train service between Hua Takhe and the northern suburb of Rangsit, through Bangkok and the old Don Mueang Airport, for a flat fare of 30 baht (less than US$1). This train connects with the Bangkok Transit System (BTS) Sky Train at Phaya Thai Station and with the Mass Rapid Transit (MRT) subway at Phetchaburi Station.

Sea. There are no regular steamship connections to Thailand, although cargo ships calling at Bangkok's Khlong Toei Port may occasionally have passenger facilities. Cruise liners call at two modern deep-sea ports: Laem Chabang, between Bangkok and Pattaya, and the island resort of Phuket. Contact a local travel agent for details.

Bus. Domestic bus service connects Bangkok and all the provinces, offering travelers standard air-conditioned coaches or VIP air-conditioned coaches serving refreshments. Bangkok's three major terminals are the Northern (Mo Chit) Bus Terminal, Southern (Sai Tai Mai) Bus Terminal, and Eastern (Ekamai) Bus Terminal. Bookings can be made through hotels and travel agents.

Car rental and chauffeur service. Travelers with a valid driver's license can rent a car. English-language road signs and maps are commonplace. International car rental companies, such as Avis, Hertz, and Budget, operate in Bangkok, Chiang Mai, Hat Yai, Pattaya, Phuket, and the island of Samui. The *Bangkok Yellow Pages* lists local car rental companies as well. Chauffeur-driven automobiles are also widely available.

Getting Around in Bangkok

Bus. Buses are numerous, ubiquitous, inexpensive, and the most common method of transport among the Thais. A bus route map can be obtained from most hotels, bookshops, and tourist information offices.

Taxi. Colorful metered taxis are easily spotted and hailed everywhere in Bangkok. The set fare is 35 baht (about US$1) for the first 2 miles (roughly 3 kilometers), then approximately 5 baht for every additional two-thirds of a mile (roughly 1 kilometer). Make sure the meter is on at the start of your journey, so there won't be any need for guesswork at the end. Passengers must pay the tolls on expressways. It's always a good idea to have your destination written in Thai—your hotel or hospital staff will be happy to write place names for you.

Tuk tuk. The famous *tuk tuk*, a three-wheeled mini taxi with open-air seating, is a fun choice for tourists. It's cheaper than a taxi and suitable for short journeys—but it's not recommended if you are in pain or healing from a medical procedure. If you end up wanting to try one anyway, remember to negotiate the fare before the ride begins.

Motorcycle taxi. Clusters of motorcyclists in numbered orange vests are based at appointed street corners, and they can speed travelers to a destination faster than any other means of transport, but a motorcycle taxi ride is not for the faint-hearted. You must wear a helmet—it's against the law to ride a motorcycle without one—but don't expect the driver to have a spare. Negotiate the fare beforehand.

Sky Train. This light elevated railway is one of the quickest and most convenient ways to travel in Bangkok. Two BTS Sky Train lines, Sukhumvit and Silom, run every few minutes from 0600 to 2400 hours daily. Fares are 15–40 baht (less than US$1.20) per journey, and day and long-term passes are available, as are free maps. (Make sure to retain your pass, as you'll need it to exit the station.) Rush-hour trains can be very cramped, especially heading toward the line intersection at Siam Central—avoid traveling at peak times if you can. The stations are usually reached by stairs or escalators (escalators only go up, but more are being added), and occasionally by elevators. Several stations have BTS Tourist Information Centers, open daily from 0800 to 2000 hours and staffed by English-speaking attendants. For more information, see www.bts.co.th.

Metro. An alternative means of traveling in Bangkok is the MRT metro. This underground train runs daily from 0600 to 2400 hours and intersects with the BTS Sky Train at three stations. Fares are 16–41 baht (less than US$1.20). One-day, three-day, and 30-day metro passes are available. For more information, see www.bangkokmetro.co.th.

Airport Rail Link. Suvarnabhumi International Airport will be connected with downtown Bangkok by a high-speed Airport Rail Link in late 2009. This link will connect to the BTS Sky Train at Phaya Thai Station and the MRT Blue Line at Phetchaburi Station.

River taxi. Many of Bangkok's major tourist attractions lie along the Chao Phraya River, making river taxis another inexpensive, fast, and enjoyable way to travel around the city. Long-tail boats can take visitors on a two-hour tour of the city's canal network for about 500 baht (less than US$15). Ferries cross the river between Bangkok and Thonburi at various points. Major riverside hotels also provide their own shuttle services.

Embassies and Consulates

It's a good idea to take with you information on the location and telephone number of your nation's embassy or consulate. You may need to contact their offices in Bangkok should you lose a passport or encounter some other difficulty while in Thailand. Here are a few of the offices typically contacted by travelers from English-speaking countries:

- Australian Embassy   66 2 287.2680
  37 Sathon Tai Road
  Thungmahamek, Sathon
  Bangkok 10120

- Canadian Embassy   66 2 636.0540
  Abdulrahim Place, 15th Floor
  990 Rama 4 Road
  Bangrak
  Bangkok 10500

- New Zealand Embassy   66 2 254.2530
  M Thai Tower, 14th Floor
  All Seasons Place
  87 Witthayu Road
  Lumphini, Pathumwan
  Bangkok 10330

- United Kingdom–British Embassy   66 2 305.8333
  1031 Witthayu Road
  Lumphini, Pathumwan
  Bangkok 10330

- United States Embassy   66 2 205.4000
  120–122 Witthayu Road
  Lumphini, Pathumwan
  Bangkok 10330

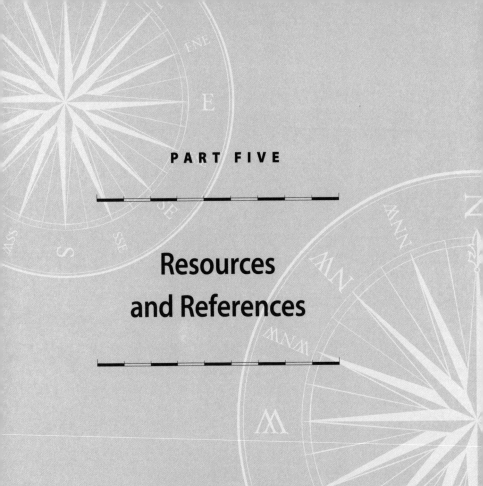

PART FIVE

Resources
and References

ADDITIONAL RESOURCES

Other Editions of *Patients Beyond Borders*

The international *Patients Beyond Borders: Second Edition* explores medical travel's practical and personal considerations and provides information on the specialties, hospitals, and accommodations currently offered to medical travelers in 21 countries. Each year Healthy Travel Media also publishes new, specialized editions of *Patients Beyond Borders*. Country-specific editions include India, Korea, Malaysia, Singapore, Taiwan, and Turkey. Visit www.patients beyondborders.com to check on special editions for your destination.

World, Country, and City Information

The World Factbook. Compiled by the US Central Intelligence Agency (CIA) and cataloged by country, this is an excellent source of general, up-to-date information about the geography, economy, and history of countries around the world. Go to www.cia.gov, find "Library and Reference" in the left column, and click on "The World Factbook."

Lonely Planet. Lonely Planet's books are arguably the most comprehensive and reliable guides for both budget and luxury travelers. The series covers every country and city destination featured in *Patients Beyond Borders*. Increasingly, its published information is being posted online as well, at www.lonelyplanet.com.

Becoming Informed Here and Abroad

You: The Smart Patient: An Insider's Guide for Getting the Best Treatment. Physicians Michael F. Roizen and Mehmet C. Oz have written a witty, often irreverent, and highly useful guide to becoming an informed patient, whether in your doctor's office or dentist's chair, on the surgeon's table, or in an emergency room. This 400-page consumer bible is packed with information on patients' rights, surgical precautions, second and third opinions, health insurance plans, health records, and precautionary advice that falls outside the scope of this book.

World Travel Guide. The publishers of the *Columbus World Travel Guide* also sponsor www.worldtravelguide.net, which offers good information on countries and major metropolitan areas throughout the world. Go to the Web site's "Choose Guide" search to find information on airports, tours, attractions, cruises, and more.

Google Earth. If you've not downloaded Google Earth, go to http://earth.google.com and do so. It's truly one of the wonders of the online world. After you follow the download instructions, you can zoom to your home's rooftop or "fly" to any continent, country, or city on the planet simply by typing in the appropriate keywords. Legends include city names, roads, terrain, populated places, borders, 3-D buildings, and more.

Information about Thailand

- Tourism Authority of Thailand (TAT) official Web site, www.tourismthailand.org
- Ministry of Public Health official Web site, http://eng.moph.go.th
- Ministry of Foreign Affairs official Web site, www.mfa.go.th
- World Health Organization, "Country Health System Profile: Thailand," 2007, www.searo.who.int/LinkFiles/Thailand_Thailand_final_031005_WT.pdf
- World Health Organization, "Health Questions About 11 SEAR Countries," www.searo.who.int/LinkFiles/Country_Health_System_Profile_10-thailand.pdf
- "Thai Traditional Medicine," http://thaifloriade.doae.go.th/hort_cd/html/frame.html

- Ministry of Public Health, *Thailand Health Profile 2001-2004,* www.moph.go.th/ops/health_48/index_eng.htm
- Adrian Towse et al., "Learning from Thailand's Health Reforms," *British Medical Journal* (2004) 328:103–105.
- Robert L. Williams et al., "Family Practice in Thailand: Will It Work?" *Journal of the American Board of Family Medicine* (January–February 2002) 15(1):73–76.
- "Research and Markets: Thailand Pharmaceuticals and Healthcare Report Q2 2008 Out Now," *Medical Letter of the CDC & FDA* (August 3, 2008):78+.

Passports and Visas

Travisa. Dozens of online agencies offer visa services—but we've found this agency, at www.travisa.com, to be reliable and accessible by telephone as well. Travisa offers good customer service and followup. Their Web site also carries links to information on immunization requirements, travel warnings, current weather, and more.

Currency Converter

www.xe.com. To learn quickly how much your money is worth in your country of interest, go to this site and click on "Quick Currency Converter."

Traveler's Tips

Smart Packing by Susan Foster (Third Edition, Smart Travel Press, 2008) includes timely information on airport security, airline regulations, and travel security. It offers advice on luggage selection, matching clothes to the occasion, and finding the right fabrics and styles for every season. The book also includes chapters on how to travel light and what to do about toiletries, cosmetics, electrical appliances, and travel gadgets.

International Hospital Accreditation

Joint Commission International (JCI). Mentioned frequently throughout this book, JCI remains the only game in town for international hospital accreditation. To see a current list of accredited hospitals by country, go to www.joint commissioninternational.org.

Medical Information

MedlinePlus is a US government–sponsored site that brings together a wealth of information from such sources as the National Library of Medicine (the world's largest medical library), the National Institutes of Health, *Merriam-Webster's Medical Dictionary* (see below), and the *United States Pharmacopeia*. Go to http://medlineplus.gov and click on any of the choices in the left column. The online tour at www.nlm.nih.gov/medline plus/tour/medlineplustour.html helps you navigate this massive site.

Merriam-Webster's Medical Dictionary. If a multisyllabic medical term stumps you, don't run out and purchase an unabridged brick of a medical dictionary— several free, online medical glossaries offer more than you probably want to know on most health topics. *Merriam-Webster's Medical Dictionary* is provided on a number of sites, including MedlinePlus (see above) and InteliHealth (www .intelihealth.com). The simplest access is through http://dictionary.reference.com.

Just type in a medical word or phrase, and voila! For a richer exploration, MedicineNet (www.medicinenet.com) and similar sources offer articles, services, and a thicket of sponsored links.

Spa Information

Check your library, bookstore, or favorite online outlet for a guide to spas. We especially like the following:

- Bernard Burt and Pamela Price. *Insiders' Guide: 100 Best Spas of the World.* Guilford, CT: Insiders' Guide, 2006.
- Judy Chapman. *Ultimate Spa: Asia's Best Spas and Spa Treatments.* Hong Kong: Periplus, 2006.
- *Wellness: Live and Retreat in the Land of Health Smiles.* Bangkok: Unseen Planet, 2008.

Medical Travel Resources

World Health Organization (WHO). On its official Web site at www.who .int, WHO provides profiles of member countries, overviews of significant health topics, and statistics of interest to health travelers and medical professional worldwide.

Medical Nomad. A group of medical professionals, technology geeks, and consultants established www.medical nomad.com in 2004 to bring together an impressive body of information, including specific data on treatments, clinics, physicians, accreditation, and other topics of interest to the health traveler. Medical Nomad's extensive database allows readers to search by procedure, provider, and destination, with clinic and country summaries as well as lay summaries of common treatments.

RevaHealth is a searchable database of healthcare providers around the world. At www.revahealth.com, the unique directory system and powerful search engine allow patients to find detailed information easily. For example, RevaHealth has a long list of heart clinics in Thailand at www.revahealth.com/coronary-vascular/thailand. The platform also lets patients select providers and talk to them directly for a consultation.

International Society of Travel Medicine (ISTM). If you're looking for information about immunizations, infectious diseases, or other aspects of medical travel, check out the ISTM Web site at www.istm.org. This organization maintains offices in Georgia, US, and in Munich, Germany, to promote safe and healthy travel and to facilitate education, service, and research activities in the field of travel medicine. Most useful to the health traveler is the society's searchable database of travel medicine practitioners and clinics.

Medical Tourism Insight is a monthly online newsletter written for the medical travel industry as well as employers, benefits managers, government officials, and prospective patients. Coverage includes objective and timely information on overseas medical care and related issues, such as health insurance and employee health benefits. The Web site is www.medicaltourisminsight.com.

International Medical Travel Journal (IMTJ). IMTJ is the world's leading journal for the medical travel industry. While geared more toward industry professionals than consumers, it does provide a free online guide for potential patients at

www.imtjonline.com. There's a free email newsletter, too, and a paid subscription service for those who are serious about industry news.

International Medical Travel Association (IMTA). Based in Singapore, IMTA and its small but growing membership advocate international patients' rights, quality-assurance standards for international hospitals, excellence in continuity of care, and other patient-provider issues. For more information, visit www.intlmta.org.

Beauty from Afar. If you're seeking more specialized information on cosmetic/aesthetic surgery or dental care, author and medical traveler Jeff Schult can fill you in on the main destinations, leading clinics and facilities, and third-party agents. Published in 2006 (Stewart, Tabori & Chang), this 224-page paperback is written in an anecdotal style, providing numerous firsthand accounts that give prospective patients a thorough perspective on the health travel experience.

Medical Tourism in Developing Countries, by Milica Z. Bookman and Karla R. Bookman (Palgrave Macmillan, 2007), explores the international marketplace for medical services and its potential for developing countries. While it's more an academic work than a consumer guide, physicians, administrators, and healthcare officials will find this book's economic perspective and vast bank of data on the industry instructive.

A couple of magazine articles are worth a trip to your local library or an online search to dig up. If you're considering in vitro fertilization, you need to read "How

Far Would You Go to Have a Baby?" by Brian Alexander, which appeared in the May 2005 issue of *Glamour*. On broader topics, Jennifer Wolff's "Passport to Cheaper Health Care?" assesses the pros and cons of medical travel. You'll find it in the October 2007 issue of *Good Housekeeping* or online at www.good housekeeping.com.

Refining Your Internet Research

*T**he Google Guide.*** While you may not wish to become a wild-eyed expert on the nuances of search engines, a little additional knowledge can greatly enhance your efficiency in narrowing your health travel choices. Consultant and Internet search guru Nancy Blachman (coauthor of *How to Do Everything with Google*) has posted a useful online tutorial entitled "The Google Guide." Go to www.googleguide.com, click on "Novice," and you'll find a wealth of information on conducting Internet searches that will greatly improve your online health travel quests. Most of this information applies to other search engines as well, including Yahoo, MSN, and AOL.

MEDICAL GLOSSARY

Many medical terms are used in this book. The following is a list of the most commonly used terms. For further information, please consult your doctor.

Acute-care. Providing emergency services and general medical and surgical treatment for sudden severe disorders (as compared with long-term care for chronic illness).

Addiction. Occurs when a person has no control over the use of a substance, such as drugs or alcohol. Also includes addictions to food, gambling, and sex.

Aesthetics. A general term for medical treatments and surgical procedures undertaken to improve appearance. Such procedures include (but are not limited to) facelifts, tummy tucks, laser resurfacing of skin, Botox injection, cosmetic dentistry, and others.

Alzheimer's disease. A degenerative disorder of neurons in the brain that disrupts thought, perception, and behavior.

Anesthesia. Loss of physical sensation produced by sedation. Anesthesia may be given as (1) general, which affects the entire body and is accompanied by loss of consciousness; (2) regional, which affects an entire area of the body; and (3) local, which affects a limited part of the body (usually superficial).

Angiography. An x-ray procedure that uses dye injected into the coronary arteries to study circulation in the heart.

Angioplasty. A procedure that uses a tiny balloon on the end of a catheter to widen blocked or constricted arteries in the heart.

Arthroscopy or arthroscopic surgery. The use of a tubelike instrument utilizing fiber optics to examine, treat, or perform surgery on a joint.

Bariatric. Pertaining to the control and treatment of obesity and allied diseases.

Birmingham hip resurfacing (BHR). A surgically implanted metal-on-metal hip joint replacement system. It is called a resurfacing prosthesis because only the surface of the femoral head (ball) is removed to implant the femoral component.

Bone densitometry. A method of measuring bone strength, used to diagnose osteoporosis.

Botox. A nonsurgical, physician-administered injection treatment to temporarily reduce moderate to severe wrinkles on the face.

Cardiac. Pertaining to the heart.

Cardiac catheterization. The insertion of a catheter into the arteries of the heart to diagnose heart disease. See also **angiography.**

Cardiothoracic. Pertaining to the heart and the chest.

Cardiovascular. Pertaining to the heart and blood vessels that make up the circulatory system. See also **vascular surgery.**

Cataract. Cloudiness of the lens in the eye, which affects vision. Cataracts, which often occur in older people, can be corrected with surgery to replace the damaged lens with an artificial plastic lens known as an intraocular lens.

Colonoscopy. An examination of the interior of the colon, using a thin, lighted tube (a colonoscope) inserted into the rectum.

Computed tomography (CT). Sometimes known as CAT scanning. A noninvasive diagnostic tool that uses x-rays to provide cross-sectional images of the body. Used to detect cancer, determine heart function, and provide images of body organs. May be used in conjunction with **positron emission tomography (PET).**

Coronary artery bypass graft (CABG). Surgical procedure to create alternative paths for blood to flow around obstructions in the coronary arteries, most often using arteries or veins from other parts of the body.

Cosmetic surgery. Plastic surgery undertaken to improve appearance. See also **aesthetics** and **plastic surgery.**

Craniofacial. Pertaining to the head and face.

CyberKnife. A tool for radiosurgery that delivers precise high-dose radiation. Can be used for tumors of the pancreas, liver, lungs, and brain.

Diabetes. A chronic disease characterized by abnormally high levels of sugar in the blood.

Discectomy. Removal of all or part of an intervertebral disc (a soft structure that acts as a shock absorber between two bones in the spine).

Electrocardiogram (EKG or ECG). A diagnostic test that measures the heart's electrical activity.

Endocrinology. The branch of medicine that studies hormonal systems and treats disorders that arise when hormones are out of balance.

Endoscope. A slender, tubular optical instrument used as a viewing system for examining an inner part of the body and, with an attached instrument, for performing surgery or detecting tumors.

Extracorporeal shock wave therapy (ESWT). A noninvasive treatment that involves delivery of shock waves to a painful area.

Gamma Knife. A form of radiation therapy that focuses low-dose gamma radiation on a precise target, such as a tumor of the brain or breast.

Gastroenterology. The branch of medicine that studies and treats disorders of the digestive system.

Genetics. The study of inheritance.

Gynecology. The branch of medicine that studies and treats females, especially pertaining to their reproductive system.

Hematology. The study of the nature, function, and diseases of the blood and of blood-forming organs.

Hemopoietic or hematopoietic. Pertaining to the formation of blood.

Hepatitis. Inflammation of the liver caused by a virus or toxin. There are different forms of viral hepatitis. Vaccines are available for hepatitis A and B. There is no vaccine for hepatitis C.

Hepatobiliary. Pertaining to the bile ducts.

Hepatology. The branch of medicine that studies and treats disorders of the liver.

Holter monitor. A wearable electronic device used to obtain a continuous recording of the heart's electrical activity. See **electrocardiogram (EKG or ECG).**

Immunization. Inoculation with a vaccine to render a person resistant to a disease.

Immunology. The branch of medicine that studies and treats disorders of the body's mechanisms for fighting disease, especially infectious diseases.

Implant. *In dentistry:* a small metal pin placed inside the jawbone to mimic the root of a tooth. Dental implants can be used to help anchor a false tooth, a crown, or a bridge. *In fertility treatment:* to place an embryo in the uterus.

Intensive Care Unit (ICU). The hospital ward in which 24-hour specialized nursing and monitoring are provided for patients who are critically ill or have undergone major surgical procedures.

International Organization for Standardization (ISO). An organization based in Geneva, Switzerland, that approves and accredits the facilities and administrations of hospitals and clinics but not their practices, procedures, or methods.

Intracytoplasmic sperm injection (ICSI). A type of fertility treatment in which a single sperm cell is inserted into an egg using special micromanipulation equipment.

Intrauterine insemination (IUI). Introduction of prepared sperm (either the male partner's or a donor's) into the uterus to improve chances of pregnancy.

In vitro fertilization (IVF). Known as the test-tube baby technique. Eggs are fertilized outside the body, and then embryos are introduced back into the woman's uterus.

Joint Commission International (JCI). The international affiliate accreditation agency of the Joint Commission. JCI inspects and accredits healthcare providers worldwide using US-based standards.

Laparoscope. A thin, lighted tube used to examine and treat tissues and organs inside the abdomen.

LAP-BAND. An adjustable silicone band inserted laparoscopically around the upper part of the stomach, thereby reducing the stomach's food storage area and promoting weight loss.

LASIK (laser-assisted *in situ* keratomileusis). A laser procedure to reduce dependency on eyeglasses or contact lenses by permanently changing the shape of the cornea, the clear covering of the front of the eye.

Liposuction. The surgical withdrawal of fat from under the skin, using a small incision and suctioning.

Lithotripsy. A procedure that breaks up kidney stones or gallstones using sound waves. Also called extracorporeal shock wave lithotripsy (ESWL).

Magnetic resonance imaging (MRI). A noninvasive diagnostic tool that uses a large magnet, radio waves, and a computer to produce clear images of the interior of the body. Used to diagnose spine and joint problems, heart disease, and cancer.

Mammography. X-ray imaging of the breast for detection of cancer.

Maxillofacial. Pertaining to the jaws and face.

Microsurgical epididymal sperm aspiration (MESA). Obtaining immature sperm cells from the epididymis (which joins the testicle to the vas deferens), in cases where obstruction in the genital tract leads to absence of sperm in the ejaculate. The recovered sperm can be used for **intracytoplasmic sperm injection (ICSI)**.

Minimal access surgery. Also called minimally invasive surgery. Any of a variety of approaches used to reduce the trauma of surgery and to speed recovery. These approaches include "keyhole" surgery, endoscopy, arthroscopy, laparoscopy, or the use of small incisions.

Myocardial infarction (MI). Heart attack.

Neonatology. The branch of medicine specializing in the care and treatment of newborns.

Nephrology. The branch of medicine that studies and treats disorders of the kidneys.

Neurology. The branch of medicine that studies and treats disorders of the nervous system, including the brain.

Neuro-oncology. The branch of medicine that studies and treats cancers of the nervous system.

Neuro-ophthalmology. The branch of medicine that studies and treats disorders of the nerves in the eye.

Neurosurgery. Surgery on the brain or other parts of the nervous system.

Obstetrics. The branch of medicine focusing on pregnancy and childbirth.

Oncology. The branch of medicine that studies and treats cancer.

Ophthalmology. The branch of medicine that studies and treats disorders of the eye.

Orthodontics. The branch of dentistry focusing on the prevention and correction of irregular tooth positioning, as by means of braces.

Orthopedics. The branch of medicine that studies and treats diseases and injuries of the bones and joints.

Osteoporosis. Thinning of the bones and reduction in bone mass, which increases the risk of fractures and decreases mobility, especially in the elderly.

Otorhinolaryngology. The branch of medicine that studies and treats ear, nose, and throat disorders.

Pacemaker. An electronic device surgically implanted into a patient's chest to regulate the heartbeat.

Parkinson's disease. A brain disorder that produces movement difficulties, most commonly among the elderly.

Pathology. The branch of medicine focusing on the laboratory-based study of disease in cells and tissues, as opposed to clinical examination of symptoms.

Pediatric. Pertaining to children.

Periodontics. The branch of dentistry focusing on the study and treatment of diseases of the bones, connective tissues, and gums surrounding and supporting the teeth.

Physiotherapy or physical therapy. The treatment or management of physical disability, malfunction, or pain by exercise, massage, hydrotherapy, and other techniques without the use of drugs, surgery, or radiation.

Plastic surgery. The branch of medicine focusing on corrective operations to the face, head, and body to restore function and (sometimes) to improve appearance (also called **cosmetic surgery**).

Polio (poliomyelitis). A paralyzing disease caused by a virus and characterized by inflammation of the motor neurons of the brainstem and spinal cord.

Positron emission tomography (PET). Also known as PET imaging or PET scanning. A diagnostic tool that captures images of the interior of the body by detecting positrons or tiny particles from radioactive material. Used to detect cancer and determine heart function; used most recently as an early clue to Alzheimer's. May be used in conjunction with **computed tomography (CT)**.

Prosthodontics. The branch of dentistry focusing on replacing missing teeth and other oral structures with artificial devices.

Psychiatry. The branch of medicine that studies and treats mental disorders.

Radiofrequency ablation (RFA). The use of electrodes to generate heat and destroy abnormal tissue.

Radiology. The branch of medicine focusing on capturing and interpreting images, such as x-rays, CT scans, and MRI scans.

Radiosurgery. The use of ionizing radiation, either from an external source (such as an x-ray machine) or an implant, to destroy cancerous or diseased tissue.

Radiotherapy. Treatment of disease with radiation, especially by selective irradiation with x-rays or other ionizing radiation or by ingestion or implantation of radioisotopes.

Reconstructive surgery. The branch of surgery focusing on the repair or replacement of malformed, injured, or lost organs or tissues of the body, chiefly by the transplant of living tissues.

Rehabilitation. The process of restoring health and improving functioning.

Renal. Pertaining to the kidneys.

Rheumatology. The branch of medicine that studies and treats disorders characterized by pain and stiffness afflicting the extremities or back.

Stem cell. An unspecialized or undifferentiated cell that can become specialized to perform the functions of diverse tissues in the body.

Stent. A tube inserted into a blood vessel or duct to keep it open. Stents are sometimes inserted into narrowed coronary arteries to help keep them open after balloon angioplasty.

Tertiary-care. Providing care of a highly specialized nature.

Testicular epididymal sperm aspiration (TESA). A surgical procedure to obtain sperm from within the testicular tissue.

Transplant. *Organ transplant:* the surgical insertion of an organ from a donor (living or deceased) into a patient to replace an organ that is diseased or malfunctioning; transplants are available for heart, liver, lungs, pancreas, kidney, cornea, and some other organs. *Stem cell transplant:* a procedure in which stem cells are collected from the blood of the patient (autologous) or a matched donor (allogeneic) and then reinserted into the patient to rebuild the immune system. *Bone marrow transplant (BMT):* a procedure that places healthy bone marrow from the patient (autograft) or a donor (allograft) into a patient whose bone marrow is damaged or malfunctioning.

Typhoid. An infectious, potentially fatal intestinal disease caused by bacteria and usually transmitted in food or water.

Ultrasound. The use of high-frequency sound waves in therapy or diagnostics, as in the deep-heat treatment of a joint or in the imaging of internal structures.

Urology. The branch of medicine that studies and treats urinary tract infections (UTIs) and other disorders of the urinary system.

Vascular surgery. The branch of medicine focusing on the diagnosis and surgical treatment of disorders of the blood vessels, excluding the heart, lungs, and brain.

Wellness. An area of preventive medicine that promotes health and well-being though various means, such as diet, exercise, yoga, tai chi, social support, and more.

X-rays. A form of electromagnetic radiation, similar to light but of shorter wavelength, which can penetrate solids; used for imaging solid structures inside the body.

INDEX

Hospital names and specialist groups are indexed in **bold**. Main treatment categories are indexed in *italics*; specific treatments may be found in the text.

A

abdominal surgery
  Vejthani Hospital, 121–123
accommodations, 16, 24
accreditation, 44, 46–47, 75, 221
activities, visitor, 200–205
acupressure
  Bangkok Hospital Medical Center,
    80–85
acupuncture. See also Chinese medicine
  Bangkok Adventist Hospital, 76–78
  Bangkok Hospital Medical Center,
    80–85
  Yanhee International Hospital,
    124–125
adolescent medicine
  Samitivej Srinakarin Children's Hospital, 119–121
advance deposits, 40–41
Adventist Healthcare Network, 76
aesthetic treatment. See also skin treatment
  Bangkok Hospital Medical Center,
    80–85
  Bangkok Hospital Phuket, 126–128
  Piyavate International Hospital,
    100–103
  Preecha Aesthetic Institute, 107–109
  Yanhee International Hospital,
    124–125
airfare, 22
airport rail link, 214
airport tax, 23, 209
airport transportation, 23–24
air transportation, 212
alcohol, 59

Alexander, Brian, 222–223
allergy treatment
  Bangkok Adventist Hospital, 76–78
  Bangkok Hospital Medical Center,
    80–85
  Bangkok Hospital Phuket, 126–128
  Bumrungrad International Hospital,
    91–96
  Phuket International Hospital,
    129–131
  Phyathai Group, 97–100
  Praram 9 Hospital, 104–106
  Samitivej Srinakarin Children's Hospital, 119–121
"all-in-one" package deals, 40
alternative medicine. See Chinese medicine; traditional medicine
alternatives to JCI, 47
Ananda Spa, 151–153
Ancient City, 202
animal life, 203–204
antiaging treatment
  Bangkok Hospital Medical Center,
    80–85
  Piyavate International Hospital,
    100–103
anticoagulant, 58
arbitration, 28
art and architecture, 202–203
arthritis. See bone and joint disorders; rheumatology
Arts of the Kingdom Museum, 202
Arusaya Spa, 186–187
assisted reproduction. See fertility/ infertility treatment; in vitro fertilization (IVF)
asthma treatment
  Bangkok Hospital Medical Center,
    80–85
  Praram 9 Hospital, 104–106
  Samitivej Srinakarin Children's Hospital, 119–121
ATMs, 209–210
audiology. See hearing treatment
Australian Council of Healthcare Standards, 47

ABOUT THE AUTHOR

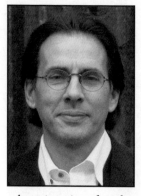

As president of Healthy Travel Media and author of *Patients Beyond Borders,* **Josef Woodman** has spent more than three years touring more than 140 medical facilities in 22 countries, researching contemporary medical tourism. As cofounder of MyDailyHealth and Ventana Communications, Woodman's pioneering background in health, wellness, and Web technology has allowed him to compile a wealth of information about global health travel, telemedicine, and new developments in consumer and institutional medical care. A noted consumer advocate for the globalization of healthcare, Woodman has lectured at Harvard Medical School and the UCLA School of Public Health, and has hosted more than a dozen seminars and workshops around the world on the topics of medical tourism and health travel.